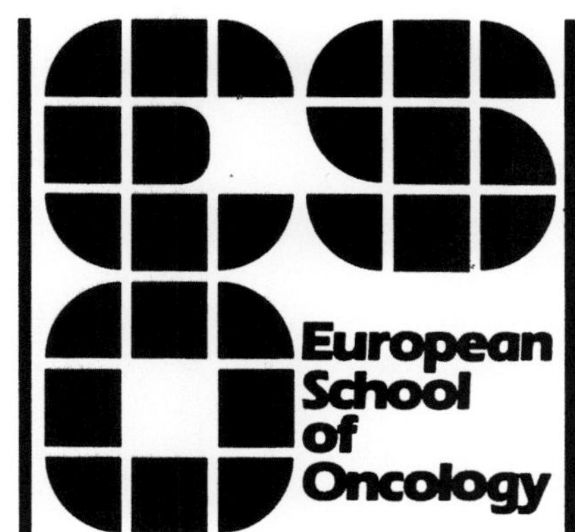

Monographs

Series Editor: U. Veronesi

F. Cavalli (Ed.)

Endocrine Therapy of Breast Cancer III

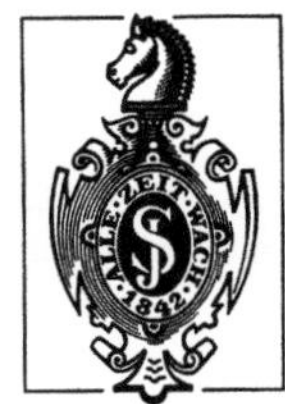

Springer-Verlag Berlin Heidelberg New York
London Paris Tokyo

Franco Cavalli

Division of Oncology, Ospedale San Giovanni,
6500 Bellinzona, Switzerland

The European School of Oncology gratefully acknowledges sponsorship for the Task Force received from

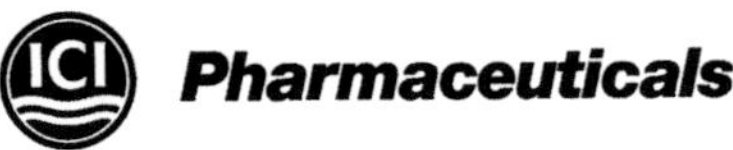

ISBN-13:978-3-642-74506-5   e-ISBN-13:978-3-642-74504-1
DOI: 10.1007/978-3-642-74504-1

Foreword

The European School of Oncology came into existence to respond to a need for information, education and training in the field of the diagnosis and treatment of cancer. There are two main reasons why such an initiative was considered necessary. Firstly, the teaching of oncology requires a rigorously multidisciplinary approach which is difficult for the Universities to put into practice since their system is mainly disciplinary orientated. Secondly, the rate of technological development that impinges on the diagnosis and treatment of cancer has been so rapid that it is not an easy task for medical faculties to adapt their curricula flexibly.

With its residential courses for organ pathologies and the seminars on new techniques (laser, monoclonal antibodies, imaging techniques etc.) or on the principal therapeutic controversies (conservative or mutilating surgery, primary or adjuvant chemotherapy, radiotherapy alone or integrated), it is the ambition of the European School of Oncology to fill a cultural and scientific gap and, thereby, create a bridge between the University and Industry and between these two and daily medical practice.

One of the more recent initiatives of ESO has been the institution of permanent study groups, also called task forces, where a limited number of leading experts are invited to meet once a year with the aim of defining the state of the art and possibly reaching a consensus on future developments in specific fields of oncology.

The ESO Monograph series was designed with the specific purpose of disseminating the results of these study group meetings, and providing concise and updated reviews of the topic discussed.

It was decided to keep the layout relatively simple, in order to restrict the costs and make the monographs available in the shortest possible time, thus overcoming a common problem in medical literature: that of the material being outdated even before publication.

UMBERTO VERONESI
Chairman, Scientific Committee
European School of Oncology

Table of Contents

Introduction

F. Cavalli

Division of Oncology, Ospedale San Giovanni, 6500 Bellinzona, Switzerland

This is the third issue of our Monograph on Endocrine Therapy of Breast Cancer. Even if it still has to become a routine, we are no longer pioneers. The many positive comments that we have received following the appearance of the first and second volumes should help us to avoid the danger of starting to consider our endeavour a routine task which has to be completed once a year. I am convinced that this third volume is of high quality and that our undertaking continues to produce a wealth of provocative thoughts and imaginative approaches.

This year we devoted our meeting to three main topics. The first is natural and acquired resistance. This is currently a topic of paramount interest to clinicians and basic researchers. Dr. King gives in his chapter a very provocative view concerning progression from steroid-responsive to unresponsive states in breast cancer. Dr. Saez looks at the same problem from a more pharmacological point of view, while Dr. Jordan highlights once more the importance of understanding resistance to antioestrogen therapy for the future comprehension of the biology of this disease.

The second topic is related to adjuvant treatment. The team Goldhirsch/Gelber this time focuses on problems related to measuring quality of life, a key issue in the never-ending discussion about adjuvant treatments. Considering the enormous excitement elicited during ASCO 1988 by the statement of the NCI concerning treatment policy in node-negative patients, the reader will undoubtedly be keen to learn which is the position taken by our group in this Monograph.

The third topic is related to new endocrine agents, with an introduction by myself on new aromatase inhibitors.

Last but not least: a remark on our second volume. There we took an unorthodox and provocative stand in relation to the results achieved in the treatment of metastatic breast cancer. A few months later a similar attitude was presented in an editorial of the most important American journal on oncology [1]: Europe is not always coming second!

Our next meeting is planned for Autumn 1989, where we shall proceed with our efforts towards a critical review of important matters in this controversial field. In the meantime, we hope to receive some useful and interesting feedback from our readers.

REFERENCE

1   Hayes DF, Henderson JC: CAF in metastatic breast cancer: Standard therapy or another effective regimen? J Clin Oncol 1987 (5):1497-1498

Progression from Steroid Responsive to Unresponsive State in Breast Cancer

R.J.B. King and P.D. Dabre

Hormone Biochemistry and Cellular Endocrinology Laboratories, Imperial Cancer Research Fund, Lincoln's Inn Fields, London WC2A 3PX, United Kingdom

Introduction

For over a century we have known that some breast cancers respond to endocrine treatment whilst others are unresponsive and yet we know little about differences or even the derivation of these two classes of breast cancer. The pioneering work of Foulds [1] produced the concept of progression from responsive to unresponsive state in which he stressed that multiple pathways of progression occurred. Unresponsive tumours could be formed from responsive antecedents or directly without passing through a responsive stage. His work with pregnancy-dependent mouse mammary tumours fitted well with the clinical picture in which both responsive and unresponsive cancers can be identified at first presentation and endocrine-induced remission is almost invariably followed by relapse [2]. Additional observations that progression to the unresponsive state is a multistage process involving cell selection and different degrees of hormone sensitivity [3-5] have been helpful at the biological level but have not defined any of the underlying molecular events. Figure 1 depicts a generally accepted version of the current status of multi-pathway evolution of unresponsive tumours which will form the basis of the present discussions. This chapter will deal with data derived from cultured mammary tumour cell lines within the context of the role of steroids in the genesis of these pathways and the molecular events involved in this model. Transition from normal to neoplastic cells will not be discussed. The chapter will conclude with clinical implications of some of the points raised herein.

Role of Steroids in Tumour Progression

A widely held view is that unresponsive breast cancers are formed from dependent cells by inheritable changes that confer advantage on the former over the latter. A responsive state also occurs that does not have an absolute requirement for hormone (Fig. 2). Support for these generalizations exists. Experimental studies, mainly based on serial transplantation of tumours *in vivo*, have demonstrated the transition from responsive to unresponsive state [3-5]; clinically,

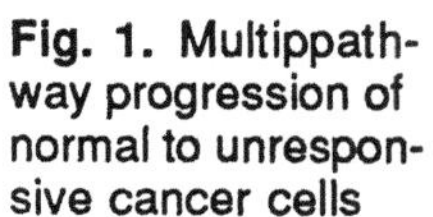

Fig. 1. Multipathway progression of normal to unresponsive cancer cells

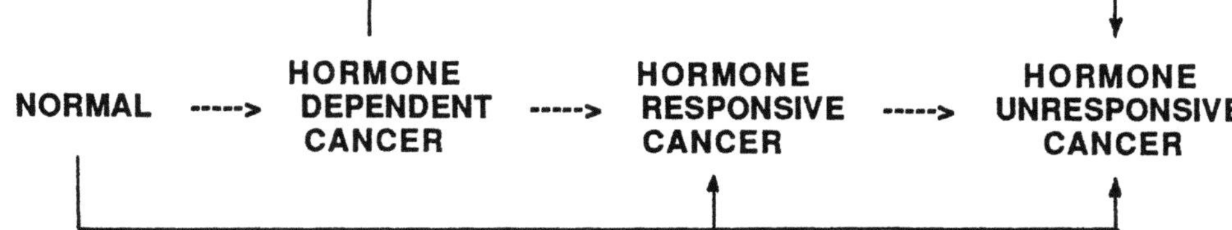

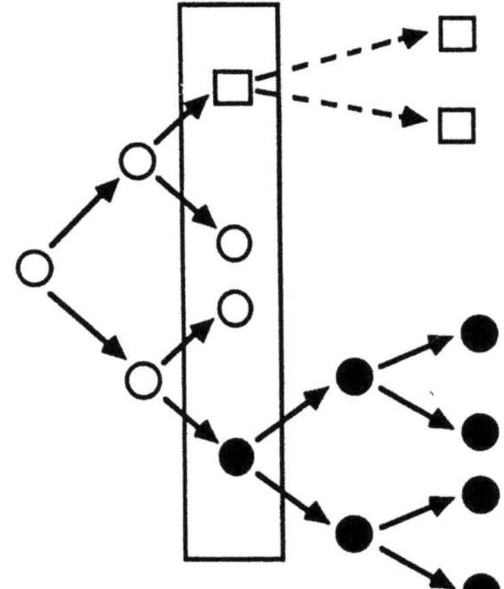

Fig. 2. Progression by cell selection. Hormone treatment stops growth of dependent cells, slows growth of responsive cells but has no effect on unresponsive cells which therefore become the predominant cell type. Adapted from reference 4

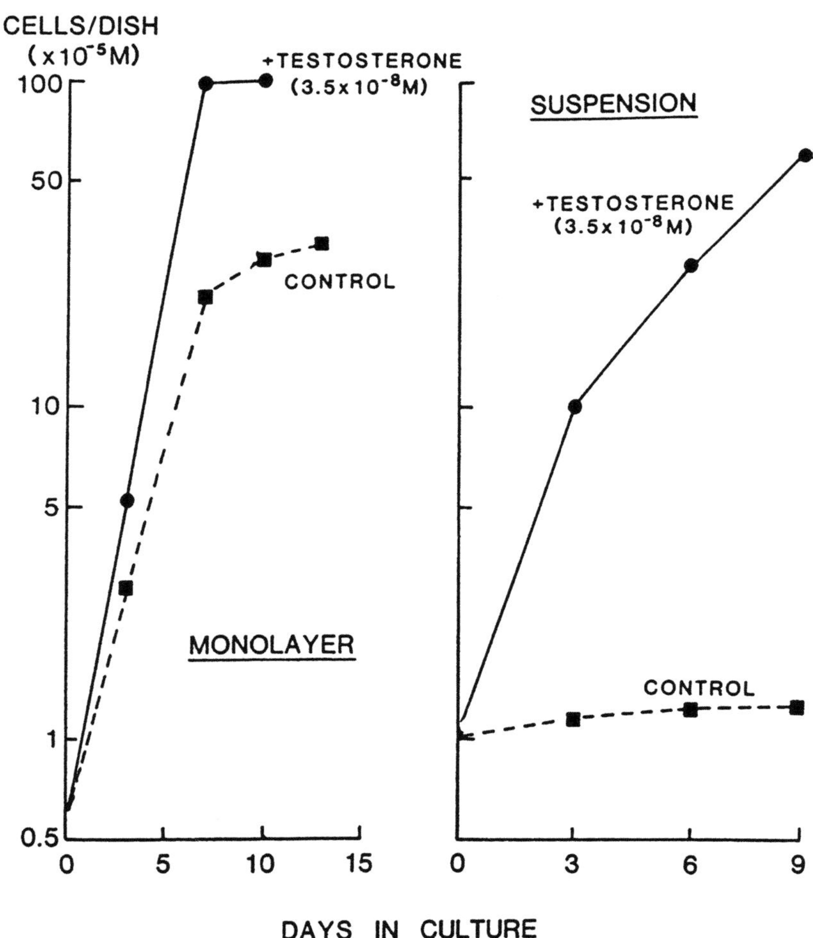

Fig. 3. Testosterone effects on S115 mouse mammary tumour cells in monolayer and suspension culture. Cells were grown either in the presence (+ testosterone) or absence (control) of androgen as monolayer (left-hand panel) or suspension (right-hand panel) cultures

hormone-induced remission followed by relapse has been ascribed to the same phenomenon. Furthermore, unresponsive tumours tend to be more active and grow faster than responsive ones [6-8]. Given the poor or non-existent mutational effect of oestrogens [9,10], there have been no suggestions that steroids could influence the initial, inheritable changes but endocrine therapy, by slowing or inhibiting growth of the responsive cells, could facilitate growth of the unresponsive population.

Cell biological studies on cultured breast tumour cells provide support for some, but not all, of the points made above. With both mouse [11,12] and human [13,14] cells, steroid withdrawal leads to the formation of unresponsive cells in an inherited manner. Thus, progression can occur in culture and be mediated (prevented) by specific steroids, a point that will be discussed later. In the mouse S115 mammary tumour system, the cells are initially androgen or glucocorticoid responsive in monolayer culture but dependent in suspension culture (Fig. 3). Progression to androgen insensitivity occurs rapidly and in a large proportion of the population [11] (Fig. 4). With human breast cancer cell lines, oestrogen deprivation can also generate populations of cells that are unresponsive for oestrogen stimulated growth (Fig. 5). Detailed comparison of loss of response in the human [13,14] and mouse [11] systems have not yet been made. Whether or not steroids other than oestrogens are protective has not been established with the human cells. Progesterone receptor is oestrogen inducible and growth is inhibited by antioestrogens in the growth-unresponsive human cells [14], which hints at differences to the murine cells.

A major feature common to both human (Fig. 5) and mouse (Fig. 4) models is that basal growth in the absence of steroid increases with no ultimate change in proliferation in the presence of hormone. Thus, loss of response apparently reflects changes in steroid-independent events, a theme that will be developed later.

In S115 cells, proliferation is regulated both by androgens and glucocorticoids paralleling the presence of their respective receptors. Most cell biological responses are similar with either class of steroid, the exception being that log-phase proliferation is stimulated by androgens and inhibited by glucocorticoids [11,15]. Importantly, unresponsiveness generated by steroid deprivation can be prevented by either androgen or glucocorticoid alone. Thus, androgens prevent loss of glucocorticoid sensitivity and glucocorticoids maintain androgen response [16]. The implication of this observation is that the presence of any functional steroid receptor complex will prevent progression. As loss of response involves well-ordered, sequential changes in several cell functions, all of which are susceptible to modulation [15,17,18], we would hypothesise that multiple genes can be switched on/off according to the steroid environment. In the mouse system, the early stages of steroid insensitivity can be reversed by readdition of steroid. However, the longer the period of deprivation, the more truncated the recovery until eventually a completely refractory state is generated [18].

The rate and extent of progression in these culture models preclude selection of unresponsive cells resulting from classical mutational events. The latter occur with a frequency of about 1 per 10^7 cell generations [19] whereas early changes in androgen sensitivity occur throughout the population of mouse cells within 20 cell doublings. The figures for oestrogen/human ZR-75 breast cancer cells are easier to define as the dependent cells do not proliferate in the absence of oestradiol and the frequency of generation of unresponsive clones is about 1 per 10^3 cells plated [20]. Several other examples of high rates of phenotypic modulation in breast [21] and other cancer [22,23] are known. Thus, mechanisms exist other than by mutation for permanently changing cell function. The term epigenetic of epimutation has been used to describe such processes [25].

Molecular Changes Associated with Loss of Response

In the previous section, the importance of elevated steroid-independent growth was emphasised but this can also be accompanied by functional changes in steroid-responsive genes. Thus, with S115 cells, induction of mouse mammary tumour virus (MMTV)

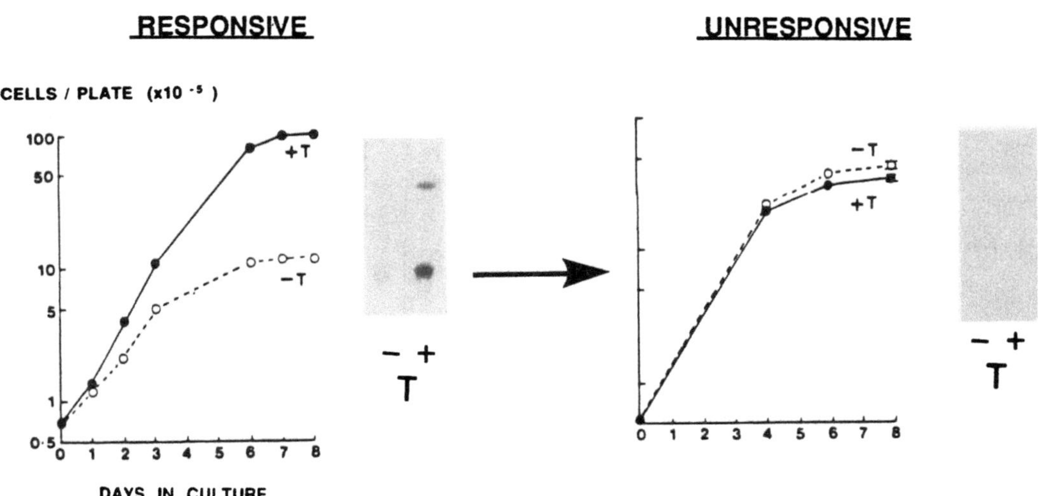

Fig. 4. Effect of long-term androgen deprivation on androgen (T) sensitivity of proliferation and specific gene expression in S115 mouse mammary tumour cells. Unresponsive cells were generated from responsive antecedents by long-term androgen withdrawal (30 weeks) and the two populations tested for short-term (1 week) sensitivity to testosterone (T). All growth responses are lost as is the regulation of a 16S mRNA transcribed from MMTV

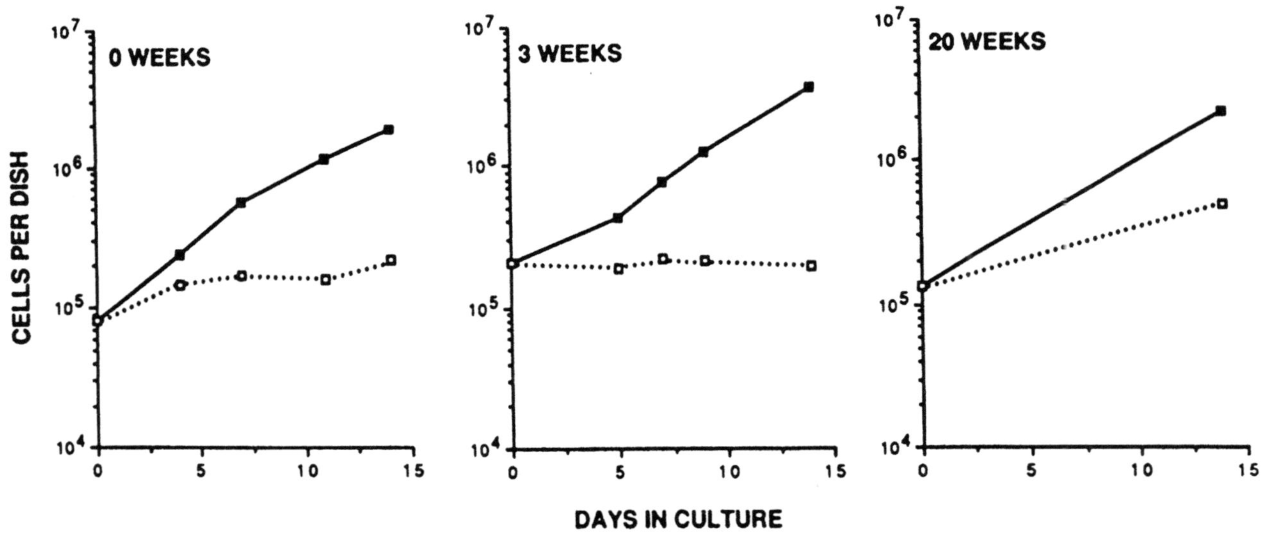

Fig. 5. Effect of long-term oestrogen deprivation on oestrogen sensitivity of proliferation in ZR-75 human breast cancer cells. Cells were maintained as monolayer cultures in steroid- and phenol red-free media for the stated number of weeks and then tested for oestradiol sensitivity in the presence (-■-) or absence (..□..) of 10^{-8} M oestradiol

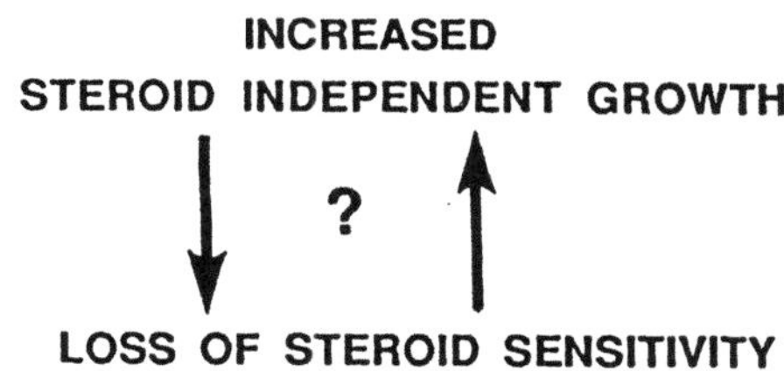

Fig. 6. Interrelationship of growth and gene expression

mRNAs is blocked (Fig. 4) at the transcriptional level [26]. Thus, two features, steroid-independent growth and steroid-inducible gene function, change as a result of steroid deprivation (Fig. 6). There is no a priori reason why these processes should be linked and further dissection of this linkage should be rewarding. What can be said with some certainty is that loss of receptor or its functionality is not involved. Transfection of a steroid-responsive marker gene into androgen receptor positive but unresponsive S115 cells clearly shows that both the androgen and glucocorticoid receptors are present and active [11,27]. MCF-7 cells that have become oestrogen-unresponsive for growth control due to prolonged oestrogen withdrawal also have functional receptors as judged from the ability of oestrogens to induce progesterone receptors [14]. Indeed, in the latter situation oestrogen receptor numbers are actually increased in the unresponsive cells.

Gene inactivation at the transcriptional level despite the presence of functional receptors could be accomplished in several ways: qualitative or quantitative changes in transcriptional or other regulatory proteins might occur as could alteration in templates with which they interact. The only data relevant to this complex situation concern DNA methylation. Hypermethylation has long been associated with gene inactivation although the cause/effect debate has not been resolved [28,29]. Furthermore, hypomethylated CG-rich regions (HTF islands) of genes that are available for regulation have been identified [30] that further implicate cytosine methylations in gene control. In S115 cells hypermethylation of cytosine residues of the MMTV genome accompanies steroid desensitisation [16,18]. In the early stage of response loss, sensitivity can be restored by readdition of steroid but

longer periods of steroid withdrawal results in a permanently refractory state: hypermethylation is associated with the latter condition. These experiments were based on DNA cleavage patterns generated by the isochisomeric restriction enzymes HpAII and MsPI which do not detect all methylated bases and more detailed analyses are required. Nevertheless, additional data based on other methods support the concept of DNA methylation as a negative signal in the glucocorticoid/lymphoma cell death [31], glucocorticoid/metallothionein gene induction [32] and progesterone, or glucocorticoid receptor/MMTV steroid response element [33] models. The only major situation where DNA methylation is unequivocally known to be involved in gene suppression is X chromosome inactivation in females, but a wider role has been proposed that has attractive implications for the model proposed in this chapter [25,34]. The essence of that proposal is that methylases exist capable of modifying cytosine bases in DNA which are crucial for gene regulation and, once methylated, the changes can be passed on to daughter cells. This epigenetic phenomenon has been termed epimutation [25].

Growth Regulation in Culture

As discussed earlier (Figures 4 and 5), loss of steroid response in culture is associated with reciprocal changes in steroid-independent growth and switching off of some specific, steroid regulated genes. To understand how these two seemingly unrelated processes might be linked, we need knowledge about how growth is regulated. The autocrine/paracrine model involving growth factors has facilitated thinking in this area and specific factors such as IGF, TGF alpha and TGF beta can be regulated in breast cancer cells by steroids [35-37]. Furthermore, transition from a responsive to an unresponsive state may involve escape from steroid modulation of these factors (Fig. 7). These studies have generated great interest and effort that will be very productive. It is already clear that the concepts behind the model are important but the details remain to be established and

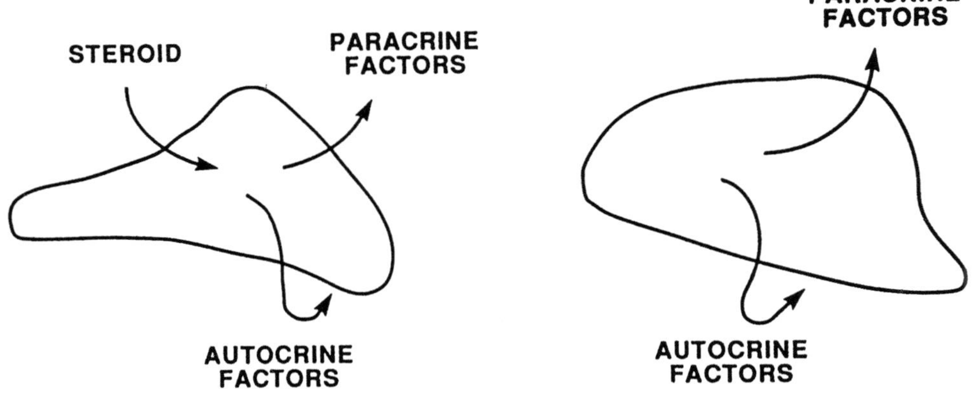

Fig. 7. Deregulation of growth factor production

are likely to be complex, involving changes in relative amounts of different factors, alterations of growth factor receptor numbers and the signal transduction pathways: novel growth factors will be identified.

At a simplistic level, one can ask the question as to whether up-regulation of a stimulatory pathway or down-regulation of inhibitory elements could best fit the loss of response model. Lack of data precludes an answer but we favour the latter for the following reason: it is not immediately obvious why an increased positive pathway, whether it be by changed production of factors such as TGF alpha or their receptors [35-37] should be linked to switching off of specific genes. If, however, the genes being blocked are involved in inhibitory pathways the linkage is understandable. Gene products have been identified that are switched off by steroid agonists or on by antagonists [38-41]. These experiments additionally illustrate an important principle that agonists such as tamoxifen can act directly by switching on specific genes as well as indirectly by blocking oestrogen response.

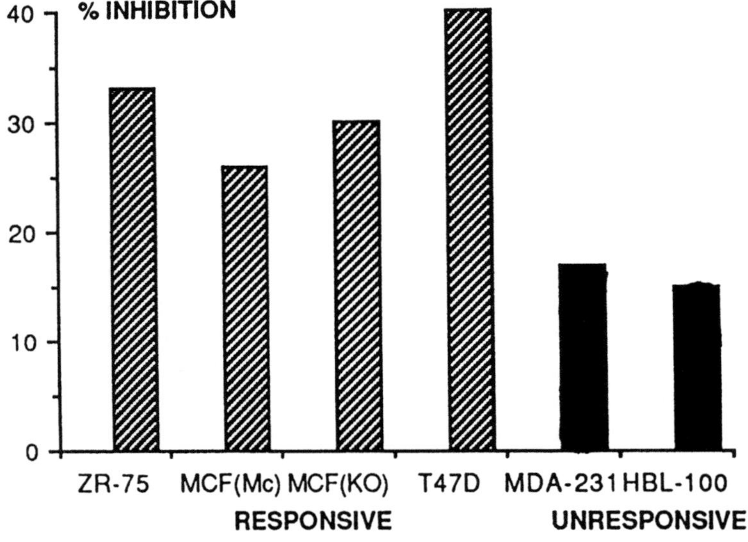

Fig. 8. Inhibition of proliferation of human breast cancer cell lines by TGFß. Monolayer cultures of the stated human breast cancer cell line were grown in steroid- and phenol red-free media for 10 days in the presence and absence of 2.5 nM TGFß

What negative pathway might be involved? At the general level one can suggest that differentiation is a negative index of growth so that the switching off of differentiation functions (dedifferentiation) would be accompanied by increased growth. This concept is compatible with the clinical data [42] on steroid sensitivity and differentiation (tumour grade). Elevated growth could be due to a general diversion of the cells' economy toward growth pathways or to more specific events; TGF beta is particularly interesting in the latter context. It is known to inhibit growth of a number of epithelial cells [43] and has therefore been categorised as a growth factor albeit in the negative sense. As more is discovered about this compound, the idea is growing that growth regulation is not its only role but induction of functions such as extracellular matrix synthesis and chemotaxis are more important; induction of cell differentiation may be its main function [44]. Thus, TGF beta production or its response pathway are candidates for loss of negative control in unresponsive cells. This avenue of speculation is worth experimental dissection and as a first step in that direction, we have been looking at the inhibitory effects of TGF beta on monolayer growth of human breast cancer cell lines (Fig. 8). These preliminary results suggest that the steroid unresponsive lines are indeed less sensitive to exogenous TGF beta than oestrogen responsive lines. In the absence of data to the contrary, the increased level of EGF (TGF alpha) receptor in unresponsive cells [45,46] could be explained by switching off an inhibitory pathway. Information on additional aspects of differentiation in responsive and unresponsive cells should be illuminating.

Model of Mammary Tumour Progression Derived from Cultured Cells

Figure 9 and Table 1 summarise the main features of our model of mammary tumour progression derived from mouse cell culture experiments with supplementary information from human cells. We would point out that it is not the only route to independence and that classical mutational events leading to cell selection can also occur [3-5].

Points 1, 2 and 4 in Table 1 have been adequately discussed in the preceding sections and elsewhere [11], whereas point 3 requires additional comment. The culture experiments indicate that absence of steroid enhances progression with no major loss in functional receptor and we have previously hypothesised [11,13] that absence of receptor as seen in either independently isolated cell lines or clinically may be a late event arising as a consequence rather that a cause of loss of sensitivity. An alternative view would be that loss of receptor, for whatever reason, would have the same end result as steroid withdrawal, namely exposure of regulatory elements of the sensitive genes to inactivation. The fact that progression by such a route has not yet been identified in culture may simply reflect our paucity of suitable experimental studies. It would be compatible with the clinical observation that metastases have a higher proportion of ER-negative tumours than do primary samples and that a limited degree of progression from positive to negative occurs within individual patients [47,48]. Similarly, paucity of data may apply to the inactivation process. Regulation of transcription is complex involving protein:DNA and protein:protein interactions and the sparse data on DNA methylation may not indicate the only defect.

Table 1. Main features of tumour progression model

---

1. Increased steroid-independent growth is accompanied by minimal change in steroid-stimulated proliferation

2. Down-regulation of genes having a negative influence on growth (dedifferentiation) may be as important as up-regulation of genes mediating positive pathways

3. Progression is driven by absence of steroid receptor complex in regulatory regions (steroid response elements) of specific genes. This could be achieved either by steroid deprivation without loss of receptor or independently by loss of functional receptor

4. One class of steroid can protect against desensitisation to another class of steroid provided the appropriate receptors are present

---

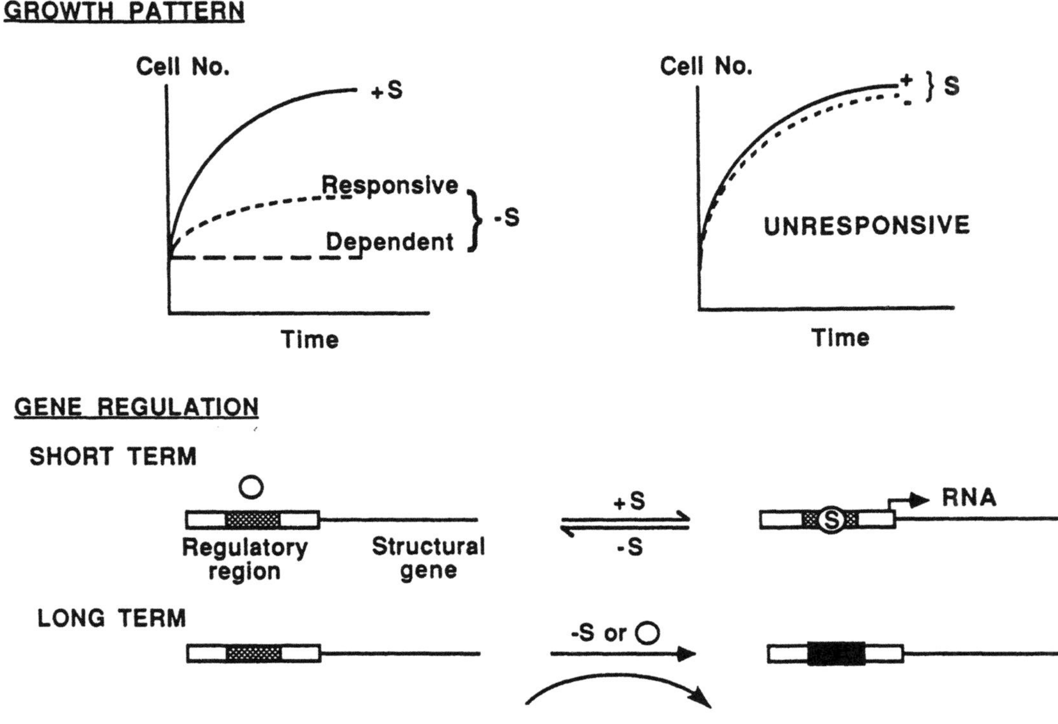

Fig. 9. Model of events involved in progression from responsive to unresponsive cells. The growth patterns of sensitive cells indicate either an absolute (dependent) or partial (responsive) requirement for steroid (S). Long-term (months) loss of either steroid or its receptor (O) leads to elevated growth in the absence of steroid. At the level of gene regulation, short-term (days) manipulation of steroid levels changes transcription via interaction of the steroid-receptor complex with specific regulatory regions (steroid response element) of the gene. Long-term (months) loss of steroid or receptor exposes this regulatory region(s) to inactivation

The fact that genes transfected into unresponsive but receptor-positive cells can lose their initial steroid sensitivity hints at a continual process of desensitisation. If confirmed by more substantial data, the concept of such a process is an important one that raises the consequential question of whether or not the process is confined to cancer cells. The only pertinent data of which we are aware relates to endometrium from postmenopausal women that can be made to mimic all the features of premenopausal endometrium by re-exposure to oestrogens and progestins [49]. This hints at differences between normal and neoplastic cells.

In the mouse system, initial loss of response can be reversed by readdition of steroid [11] but no data are available on this point for human cells. The generality or otherwise of this phenomenon should be established as it has clinical implications (see below).

Clinical Aspects

The speculative model outlined on the preceding pages has a number of clinical implications that are worth identifying.

The most useful biochemical markers of breast cancer behaviour are oestrogen and progestin receptors [50] and indices of cell proliferation such as percentage of cells in S phase, ^{3}H thymidine labelling index or mitotic activity [51]. The model described in the preceding sections should therefore be put in the context of these markers.

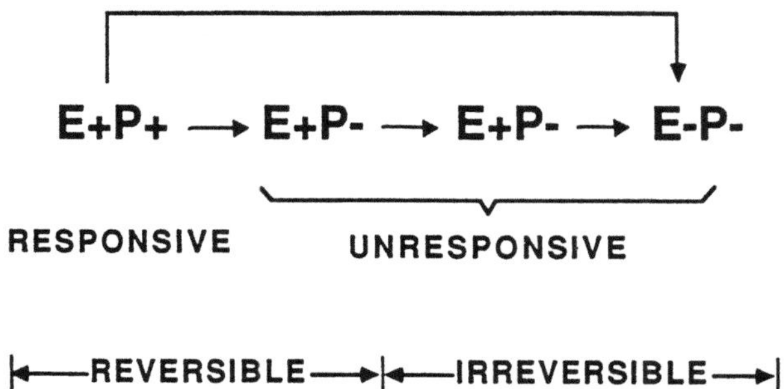

Fig. 10. Model of human breast cancer progression as indicated by receptor phenotypes. E and P = oestrogen and progestin receptor, respectively

The idea of postreceptor defects in the oestrogen response pathway led to the identification of ER+PR- tumours with a poorer response rate to hormone therapy than ER+PR+ tumours. However, neither category give ideal predictions with about one third of ER+PR+ tumours not responding whilst about a quarter of ER+PR- tumours exhibit good endocrine responses [50]. There are undoubtedly multiple explanations for these deficiencies such as cellular heterogeneity, strict criteria for defining a response and suboptimal analytical methods, but our model may help define additional biological reasons that can be exploited (Fig. 10). If there is an increasing rate of steroid-insensitive proliferation as progression occurs, then, at suboptimal steroid levels such as exist in postmenopausal women, one would predict that slower growing ER+ tumours would have a higher response rate than faster proliferating ones of similar ER phenotype. Inclusion of indices of proliferation is not a novel suggestion and supportive data exist for that prediction [51,52].

Preferential selection of unresponsive clones has long been the explanation for progression and ample data are available that it does occur [3-5]. However, it is difficult to reconcile such a mechanism with the clinical observation that a good response to a first round of endocrine therapy followed by relapse, is frequently indicative of response to a second endocrine treatment. Such behaviour might be anticipated if epigenetic mechanisms were involved and the initial stage of progression were reversible.

The age-adjusted incidence of breast cancer rises through the premenopausal years, temporarily plateaus or even falls at about the time of the menopause (Clemeson's Hook) and then resumes its rise postmenopausally. This behaviour can be explained by two-disease models in which pre- and postmenopausal breast cancers exist as different entities [53]. It is also possible that the incidence changes over the menopausal period reflect changes in growth rate of occult cancer cells and thereby changes in cancer detectability. The steroid replete premenopausal environment would promote growth of responsive cells. At the climacteric, steroid decline would have two effects, slow the growth rate and promote the generation of unresponsive cells. It is known that tumours first detected in the perimenopausal period respond poorly to hormones and have an aggressive natural history [2]. This discussion assumes a fall in biologically available levels of oestrogens at the menopause. However, endogenous oestrogens are surprisingly high, in the nanomolar range, in both breast tumours [54,55] and uteri [56] from postmenopausal women. Despite these high overall concentrations, they must be biologically inactive as, in the case of endometrium, the cells are atrophic [56]. The basis of this accumulation of oestradiol in a biologically inert state has not been established but we feel that the data on endogenous steroid levels in postmenopausal tissues do not invalidate our ideas.

Another anomaly that is explicable by our model is why oestradiol receptor has predictive value for response to all types of endocrine therapy. If one class of steroid can protect against loss of response to other classes of steroid, provided their respective receptors are present, the clinical data are understandable. The presence of oestradiol receptor would increase the probability that the tumour cells retained their sensitivity to other steroid receptor complexes.

Histochemical methods have highlighted the remarkable heterogeneity within individual human breast tumours, observations that extend to proportions of hormone-sensitive and insensitive cells within a tumour mass [57,58]. The pattern of heterogeneity does not always fit with that expected from outgrowth of clonally derived unresponsive cells. Frequently one sees numerous individual cells or small foci of cells that stain differently to the bulk of the tumour for oestradiol receptor [59], progesterone receptor [60] or oestradiol receptor-related proteins [58]. Such a pattern is compatible with epigenetic and reversible changes in individual cells and also with the data indicating that responsive and unresponsive cells within the same environment can talk to each other [61].

If hormone withdrawal actively promotes the generation of unresponsive cells then ablative surgery such as ovariectomy may not be the best form of treatment in the long term. If, however, the presence of steroid receptor complexes within the cell nucleus protect against loss of sensitivity, alternative regimes are possible. Antioestrogens might maintain the hormone sensitive state as might glucocorticoids or progestins at the same time as achieving the desired remission. If some forms of hormone insensitivity can be reverted to the sensitive state by hormones, this would support the case for additive rather that ablative treatment. It is of course possible that a combination of ablative plus additive therapy would be beneficial. Trials of ovariectomy plus glucocorticoid [62] indicate that this is the case. The efficacies of such a combined treatment are usually explained on the basis of blocking residual hormone action or pro

duction after ovariectomy but are equally compatible with our model.

An understanding of the molecular events involved in the transition from responsive to unresponsive state might indicate therapies that could prevent or even reverse that transition. For example, if our thoughts as to the role of DNA methylation are valid, prevention of methylation by drugs such as azacytidine might be tested.

Finally, where should one fit the data on elevated EGF (TGF alpha) receptor [45,46] and the related *neu* (cERB B) oncogene product [63,64] into our model? They are clearly increased in unresponsive cells and presumably there are biological sequelae to that fact. The increased EGF receptor activity is paralleled by changes in its mRNA so this up-regulation may be an example of switching off a negative regulator as described above but there are no supportive facts for that view. Gene amplification can explain some cases of increased *neu* protein [65], a change that may be independent of any of the mechanisms discussed in this chapter.

At the present time, these comments are speculative but we feel that they open novel avenues of investigation that will prove beneficial.

REFERENCES

1   Foulds L: Neoplastic Development. 1969 (1):46-90 Academic Press, London
2   Hayward J: Hormones and human breast cancer. Recent Results in Cancer Research. Springer-Verlag, Berlin 1970
3   Kim U: Factors influencing the generation of phenotypic heterogeneity in mammary tumors. In: Mihich E (ed) Biological Responses in Cancer. Plenum Press, New York 1985 pp 91-124
4   Isaacs J: Mechanisms for and implications of the development of heterogeneity of androgen sensitivity in prostatic cancer. In: Owens AH, Coffey DS and Baylin SB (eds) Tumor Cell Heterogeneity: Origins and Implications. Academic Press, New York 1982 pp 99-111
5   Matsuzawa A: Hormone dependence and independence of mammary tumours in mice. Int Rev Cytol 1986 (103):303-340
6   King RJB, Smith JA and Steggles AW: Oestrogen-binding and the hormone responsiveness of tumours. Steroidologia 1970 (I):73-88
7   Hähnel R: Steroid receptor status, tumour growth and prognosis. In: Stoll BA (ed) Endocrine Relationships in Breast Cancer. Heinemann, London 1982 pp 107-143
8   Clark GM, McGuire WL, Hubay CA, Pearson OH and Marshall JS: Progesterone receptors as a prognostic factor in stage II breast cancer. N Engl J Med 1983 (209):1343-1347
9   Ambrus JL, Gilette M, Nolan C, Jung O, Regalla-Spavento S, Spavento P, Novick A, Suchetzky C, Ambrus CM: Estrogens and endometrial cancer. In: Pasetto N, Paoletti R and Ambrus JL (eds) The Menopause and Postmenopause, MTP Press, Lancaster 1980 pp 237-244
10 IARC Monographs on the Evaluation of Carcinogenic Risk of Chemicals to Man. Vol 6: Sex Hormones. International Agency for Research on Cancer, Lyon 1974
11 Darbre PD and King RJB: Steroid hormone regulation of cultured breast cancer cells. In: Lippman ME and Dickson RB (eds): Breast Cancer: Cellular and Molecular Biology. Martinus Nijhoff, Boston 1988 pp 307-341
12 Noguchi S, Nishizawa Y, Uchida N, Yamaguchi K, Sato B, Kitamura Y and Matsumoto K: Stimulative effect of physiological doses of androgen or pharmacological doses of estrogen on growth of Shionogi carcinoma 115 in mice. Cancer Res 1985 (45):5746-5750
13 Darbre PD, Glover JF and King RJB: Effects of steroids and their antagonists on breast cancer cells: therapeutic implications. Report of SAKK Workshop, Lucerne 1987. To be published in Contributions to Oncology
14 Katzenellebogen BS, Kendra KL, Norman ML and Berthois Y: Proliferation, hormonal responsiveness and estrogen receptor content of MCF-7 human breast cancer cells grown in the short-term and long-term absence of estrogens. Cancer Res 1987 (47):4355-4360
15 Darbre PD and King RJB: Differential effects of steroid hormones on parameters of cell growth. Cancer Res 1987 (47):2937-2944
16 Darbre PD and King RJB: Interaction of different steroid hormones during progression of tumour cells to steroid autonomy. Int J Cancer 1987 (40):802-806
17 Couchman JR, Yates J, King RJB and Badley RA: Changes in microfilament and focal adhesion distribution with loss of androgen responsiveness in cultured mammary tumor cells. Cancer Res 1981 (41):263-269
18 Darbre P and King RJB: Progression to steroid autonomy in S115 mouse mammary tumour cells: role of DNA methylation. J Cell Biol 1984 (99):1410-1415
19 Baker RM: Nature and use of ouabain-resistant mutants. In: Hsie AW, O'Neill JP and McElheny VK (eds) Banbury Report 2. Mammalian Cell Mutagenesis: The Maturation of Test Systems. Cold Spring Harbor Laboratory, Cold Spring Harbor 1979 pp 237-247
20 Darbre PD: Personal communication
21 Welch DR, Evans DP, Tomasovic SP, Milas L and Nicolson GL: Multiple phenotypic divergence of mammary adenocarcinoma cell clones. Clin Expl Metastases 1984 (2):357-371
22 Fidler IJ: Review: biologic heterogeneity of cancer metastases. Breast Cancer Res Treat 1987 (9):17-26
23 Nicolson GL: The evolution of phenotypic diversity in metastatic tumor cells. In: Mihich E (ed) Biological Responses in Cancer. Plenum Press, New York 1985 pp 71-89
24 Frost P and Kerbel RS: On a possible epigenetic mechanism(s) of tumor cell heterogeneity. Cancer Metas Rev 1983 (2):375-378
25 Holliday R: The inheritance of epigenetic defects. Science 1987 (238):163-170
26 Darbre P, Page M and King RJB: Androgen regulation by the long terminal repeat of mouse mammary tumor virus. Mol Cel Biol 1986 (6):2847-2854
27 Darbre PD and King RJB: Progression to steroid insensitivity can occur irrespective of the presence of functional steroid receptors. Cell 1987 (51):521-528
28 Felsenfeld G and McGhee J: Methylation and gene control. Nature 1982 (296):602-603
29 Cedar H: DNA methylation and gene activity. Cell 1988 (53):3-4
30 Bird AP: CpG-rich islands and the function of DNA methylation. Nature 1986 (321):209-213
31 Gasson JC, Ryden T and Bourgeois S: Role of de novo DNA methylation in the glucocorticoid resistance of a T-lymphoid cell line. Nature 1983 (302):621-623
32 Compere SJ and Palmiter RD: DNA methylation controls the inducibility of the mouse metallothionein-I gene in lymphoid cells. Cell 1981 (25):233-240
33 von der Ahe D, Renoir JM, Buchou T, Baulieu EE and Beato M: Receptors for glucocorticosteroid and progesterone recognize distinct features of a DNA regulatory element. Proc Natl Acad Sci USA 1986 (83):2817-2821

34 Holliday R: X-chromosome reactivation. Nature 1987 (327):661-662

35 Lippman ME, Dickson RB, Gelmann EP, Rosen N, Knabbe C, Bates S, Valverius E, Bronzert D, Huff K and Kasid A: Human breast carcinoma cells produce growth regulatory peptides. In: Bresciani F, King RJB, Lippman ME and Raynaud JP (eds) Hormones and Cancer 3. Progress in Cancer Research and Therapy. Raven Press, New York 1988 pp 203-213

36 Dickson RB and Lippman ME: Control of human breast cancer by estrogen, growth factors and oncogenes. In: Lippman ME and Dickson RB (eds) Breast Cancer: Cellular and Molecular Biology. Martinus Nijhoff, Boston 1988 pp 119-165

37 Salomon DS and Kidwell WR: Tumor associated growth factors in malignant rodent and human mammary epithelial cells. In: Lippman ME and Dickson RB (eds) Breast Cancer: Cellular and Molecular Biology. Martinus Nijhoff, Boston 1988 pp 363-389

38 Phillips CL, Lin LW, Wu JC, Guzman K, Milsted A and Miller WL: 17ß-Estradiol and progesterone inhibit transcription of the genes encoding the subunits of ovine follicle-stimulating hormone. Mol Endo 1988 (2):641-649

39 Eastman-Reks S and Vedeckis WV: Glucocorticoid inhibition of c-*myc*, c-*myb* and c-Ki-*ras* expression in a mouse lymphoma cell line. Cancer Res 1986 (46):2457-2462

40 Knabbe C, Lippman ME, Wakefield LM, Flanders KC, Kasid A, Derynck R and Dickson RB: Evidence that transforming growth factor-ß is a hormonally regulated negative growth factor in human breast cancer cells. Cell 1987 (48):417-428

41 Rochefort H: Do antiestrogens and antiprogestins act as hormone antagonists or receptor-targeted drugs in breast cancer? TIPS 1987 (8):126-128

42 Blamey RW, Elston CW, Haybittle JL and Griffiths K: Prognosis in breast cancer: the Nottingham-Tenovus trial. In: Bulbrook RD and Taylor DJ (eds) Commentaries on Research in Breast Disease. Alan R Liss, New York 1983 (3):94-112

43 Massague J: The TGF-ß family of growth and differentiation factors. Cell 1987 (49):437-438

44 Sporn MB, Roberts AB, Wakefield LM and de Crombrugghe B: Some recent advances in the chemistry and biology of transforming growth factor-beta. J Cell Biol 1987 (105):1039-1045

45 Sainsbury JRC, Farndom JR, Needham GK, Malcolm AJ and Harris AL: Epidermal-growth-factor receptor status as predictor of early recurrence of and death from breast cancer. Lancet 1987 (1):1398-1402

46 Davidson NE, Gelmann EP, Lippman ME and Dickson RB: Epidermal growth factor receptor gene expression in estrogen receptor-positive and negative human breast cancer cell lines. Mol Endo 1987 (1):216-223

47 Mobbs BG, Fish EB, Pritchard KI, Oldfield G and Hanna WH: Estrogen and progesterone receptor content of primary and secondary breast carcinoma: influence of time and treatment. Eur J Cancer Clin Oncol 1987 (23):819-826

48 King RJB, Stewart JF, Millis RR, Rubens RD and Hayward JL: Quantitative comparison of estradiol and progesterone receptor contents of primary and metastatic human breast tumors in relation to response to endocrine treatment. Breast Cancer Res Treat 1982 (2):339-346

49 King RJB and Whitehead MI: Estrogen and progestin effects on epithelium and stroma from pre- and postmenopausal endometria: application to clinical studies of the climacteric syndrome. In: Jasonni VM, Nenci I and Flamigni C (eds) Steroids and Endometrial Cancer. Raven Press, New York 1983 pp 109-115

50 Hawkins RA, Roberts MM and Forrest APM: Oestrogen receptors and breast cancer: current status. Br J Surg 1980 (67):153-169

51 McGuire WL: Prognostic factors for recurrence and survival in human breast cancer. Breast Cancer Res Treat 1987 (10):5-9

52 Paradiso A, Lorusso V, Tommasi S, Schittulli F, Maiello E and De Lena M: Relevance of cell kinetics to hormonal response of receptor positive advanced breast cancer. Breast Cancer Res Treat 1988 (11):31-36

53 Farewell VT: Statistical methods and mathematical models for research in breast disease. In: Bulbrook RD and Taylor DJ (eds) Commentaries on Research in Breast Disease. Alan R Liss, New York 1979 (1):193-232

54 van Landeghem AAJ, Poortman J, Nabuurs M and Thijssen JHH: Endogenous concentration and subcellular distribution of estrogens in normal and malignant human breast tissue. Cancer Res 1985 (45):2900-2906

55 Fishman J, Nisselbaum JS, Menendez-Botet J and Schwartz MK: Estrone and estradiol content in human breast tumors: relationship to estradiol receptors. J Steroid Biochem 1977 (8):893-896

56 Vermeulen-Meiners C, Jaszmann LJB, Haspels AA, Poortman J and Thijssen JHH: The endogenous concentration of estradiol and estrone in normal human postmenopausal endometrium. J Steroid Biochem 1984 (21):607-612

57 Schlom J: Basic principles and applications of monoclonal antibodies in the management of carcinomas: the Richard and Hinda Rosenthal Foundation Award Lecture. Cancer Res 1986 (46):3225-3238

58 Cano A, Coffer AI, Adatia R, Mills RR, Rubens RD and King RJB: Histochemical studies with an estrogen receptor-related protein in human breast tumors. Cancer Res 1986 (46):6475-6480

59 Shimada A, Kimura S, Abe K, Nagasaki K, Adachi I, Yamaguchi K, Suzuki M, Nakajima T and Miller LS: Immunocytochemical staining of estrogen receptor in paraffin sections of human breast cancer by use of monoclonal antibody: comparison with that in frozen sections. Proc Natl Acad Sci USA 1985 (82):4803-4807

60 Perrot-Applanat M, Groyer-Picard MT, Lorenzo F, Jolivet A, Vu Hai MT, Pallud C, Spyratos F and Milgrom E: Immunocytochemical study with monoclonal antibodies to progesterone receptor in human breast tumors. Cancer Res 1987 (47):2652-2661

61 Jordan VC: Resistance to Antioestrogen Therapy: a challenge for the future. In: Cavalli F (ed) Endocrine Therapy in Breast Cancer III. European School of

Oncology Monograph Series, Springer Verlag, Heidelberg 1989 (This volume)

62 Stewart JF, Rubens RD, King RJB, Minton MJ, Steiner R, Tong D, Winter PJ, Knight RK and Hayward JL: Contribution of prednisolone to the primary endocrine treatment of advanced breast cancer. Eur J Cancer Clin Oncol 1982 (18):1307-1314

63 Slamon DJ, Clark GM, Wong SG, Levin WJ, Ullrich A, McGuire WL: Human breast cancer: correlation of relapse and survival with amplification of the HER-2/*neu* oncogene. Science 1987 (235):177-182

64 Berger MS, Locher GW, Saurer S, Gullick WJ, Waterfield MD, Groner B and Hynes NE: Correlation of *c-erb*B-2 gene amplification and protein expression in human breast carcinoma with nodal status and nuclear grading. Cancer Res 1988 (48):1238-1243

65 Venter DJ, Tuzi NL, Kumar S and Gullick WJ: Overexpression of the *c-erb*B-2 oncoprotein in human breast carcinomas: immunohistochemical assessment correlates with gene amplification. Lancet 1987 (1):69-72

Drug Resistance

S. Saez

Centre Leon Berard, 28 rue Laennec, 69373 Lyon Cedex 08, France

Normal cells and tissues are provided with selective means to protect them against endogenous substances produced in excess in the body or against toxic exogenous substances.

In the first case, a central feedback mechanism regulates any overproduction of endogenous factors, in association or not with a desensitisation process of the target cell. In the second case, the immunological system is in charge of the protection of all the cells against proteins and various toxins. Both represent general responses.

Other processes can be developed by the peripheral cells themselves to protect them against the deleterious activity of small non-immunogenic molecules of natural origin or synthetic chemical substances. In these circumstances, the cells express properties which remain latent in normal conditions. The biological changes are triggered when the cells are in contact with substances which do no mimic a physiological function. The common feature of these agents is that they are not normally introduced into the body.

While this capacity of adaptation of the tissues of the organism has not been analysed until recently, the ancients were already aware of it: it can be speculated that the experimentally induced and acquired drug resistance of Mithridates was not directed only toward toxic peptides.

The efficacity of any drug at the cell level implies that it is transferred into the cell and stays near its site of action which is specific of its biochemical and biophysical properties. To take an example, cholera toxin interferes with phosphodiesterase activity and impairs ion and water membrane exchange in the digestive mucosa. Drugs called antimetabolites act at the level of thymidine synthesis, others inhibit DNA transcription and replication by intercalation between the double strings. The toxicity may also be indirect and related to free radicals and peroxides generated by drugs and ionising radiations as well.

It has been observed that the acquired drug resistance is generally associated with a significant decrease in cellular drug accumulation. It can be supposed that resistance is achieved by various means which contribute to changes in cell permeability, alterations of the drug and/or its targets. The rise of new activities of the cells in specific circumstances is related to their genetic equipment. They become activated or overactivated whenever necessary. These processes may be reversible. They are classified into two groups:

1) Resistance specifically related to the site of action of the drug. It concerns DNA protection and repair, overproduction of targets of antimetabolites.

2) Pleiotropic resistance including a) the detoxification processes, metabolic conversion of the drugs and reduction of peroxides and free radicals; b) selective change in cell permeability.

Resistance Related to Modification of the Drug Target

Several mechanisms of resistance have been identified which counter the drug-induced inhibition of DNA synthesis. Each of these mechanisms represents the specific response of the cell to one step in the drug action pathway.

The antitumour agent **hydroxyurea** specifically inhibits DNA synthesis. Its target site of action is an enzyme, the ribonucleotide reductase which regulates the reduction of ribonucleotides into deoxyribonucleotides [1]. Hydroxyurea inhibits the action of this enzyme by interacting with one of its two subunits, the M2 component [2]. The cell responds to this effect by changes in the production of M2. An amplification of the M2 gene, initially limited, results in an increase of the M2 mRNA. In addition, a permanent high level of M2 is also provided by an increase in translational efficiency, without change in the degradation of the protein [3]. Both contribute to an increase in the amount of available enzyme.

Methotrexate belongs to the family of antifolate agents. It is a structural competitor of the folate utilising enzymes that catalyze one carbon transfer in the synthesis of purines and pyrimidines. The dihydrofolate reductase specifically transforms dihydrofolate into tetrahydrofolate. Methotrexate is a strong competitive inhibitor of this reaction.

Shimke has demonstrated the major mechanisms generating resistance to methotrexate [4]. He showed that resistant cells become able to produce enough enzyme for DNA synthesis, and overcome the activity of the inhibitor. In this example, the gene coding for the dihydrofolate reductase is amplified, leading to the overproduction of a normal enzyme. Shimke has suggested that this process is more easily generated when the mean level of inhibitor is rather low and fluctuant. Inhibition of DNA synthesis or DNA damage is followed by overreplication of the corresponding zone of DNA, which can lead to gene amplification [5,6].

DNA-**topoisomerases** are enzymes that regulate the superhelical density of DNA by transiently nicking either one (type I) or both (type II) strands of the DNA helix. It is suggested that they may be involved in many aspects of DNA metabolism including transcription, replication, recombination and chromosome segregation and mitosis [7,8]. Topoisomerase I activity is related to transcription independently of proliferation. The majority of topoisomerase I is localised in the nucleolus at the rRNA genes [9]. Topoisomerase II activity is greater in proliferating than in quiescent cells. This activity is rapidly lost upon cessation of mitotic activity in normal cells. It is considered as a specific marker of normal cell proliferation. In contrast, it is permanently maintained at a high level in transformed cells [8].

The activity of actinomycin D is related to topoisomerase I, by extending the half-life of covalent topoisomerase-DNA complex [9] while topoisomerase II is the target of many antitumour drugs, DNA intercalators and epipodophyllin. These agents inhibit topoisomerase II activity by trapping the enzyme with DNA cleavage complexes [10-12]. Their mode of action explains why they are more efficient in proliferating than quiescent cells. Inhibitors of ornithine decarboxylase, which deplete the cell polyamine content, enhance the activity of topoisomerase II-reactive drugs [13].

The acquired resistance is associated with a lower level of topoisomerase II and a reduced formation of DNA breaks [14,15]. However, this resistance is not due to the absence of topoisomerase II. It could be related to a nuclear modulating activity mediated by topoisomerase I.

Pleiotropic Resistance

Various types of drugs can be involved in a process of pleiotropic resistance. The process of resistance is, in these cases, directed towards the cell capacity for detoxication, and changes in selective permeability responsible of an accelerated efflux for the drug.

Free radicals and peroxides generated by drugs and ionising radiations contribute to their cytotoxic activity. The cell is able to react by various pathways leading to a decreased formation and/or inactivation of these radicals.

The peroxidase activity of resistant cells is enhanced and results in a marked decrease in the formation of hydroxyl radicals after exposure to drugs like adriamycin [16].

This activity is associated with that of **glutathione transferase** which contributes to the process of detoxification by another pathway: it acts by conjugating the toxic substance on the sulfur radical of cysteine molecule of glutathione.

The activity and the amount of both peroxidase and glutathione transferase are elevated in cells which have been in contact with a drug and have thereby become resistant. The increase in peroxidase activity contributes to a lowered formation of hydroxyl radicals generated by different cytotoxics (nitrogen mustard - adriamycin). Conjugation to glutathione favours the elimination of foreign chemical agents such as alkaloids, quinone, platinum [17]. In normal sensitive cells, the level of glutathione transferase is low. In previously treated tissues, its level seems to correlate with the degree of drug resistance [16,18,19]. As an example, head and neck tissues usually have a low level of enzyme. The tumours arising in this area are usually sensitive to nitrogen mustard. Conversely, tumours of the colon, lung, prostate and pancreas have a higher concentration of the enzyme and respond poorly to the treatment [20]. It is also expressed in the normal placenta [21].

The gene coding for glutathione transferase has been cloned. Investigations using Northern and Southern analysis have been carried out in a variety of normal and tumour tissues. In normal tissues its expression is at the highest level in rat liver and kidney [22]. It is usually overexpressed in resistant cells but is generally not amplified [16,19].

It is interesting to note that the same alteration of the gene function is induced in liver cells exposed to a variety of carcinogens and cytotoxics [9]. The same overexpression of glutathione transferase is observed in resistant breast cancer cells, resistant leukaemia and in rat hyperplastic liver nodules which have developed resistance to various hepatotoxins [16,23]. It is suggested that the increase in the cell capacity to conjugate the drug to glutathione plays a role in the mechanism of resistance.

Further observations are in favour of this hypothesis [24-27]. Resistant cells have a higher glutathione content than their normal counterparts [26]. Conversely, it has been shown that the thiol depletion of tumour tissue potentiates the drug's toxicity [25,27]. The reappearance of sensitivity depends upon the degree of depletion which can be achieved and on the initial level of glutathione in the tissue. In this regard, bone marrow was found to have a relatively low content in glutathione and to be the most resistant to thiol depletion

by agents like **buthionine sulfoximine**, while heart and kidney are more sensitive [27]. The differences in the initial rate of glutathione depletion reflect also its usual rate of utilisation and turnover in a given tissue. Experiments by Kramer et al. [27] indicate that tumours are usually more sensitive to buthionine sulfoximine-induced depletion than normal tissue. But the high sensitivity of tissues like the renal tissue explains that buthionine pretreatment may also enhance the renal toxicity of drugs such as MeCCNU and cis-platinum, two agents with a tendency to induce phrotoxicity [27].

Alteration of drug transport in the cell is often associated with other mechanisms of resistance which severely affect the efficacy of treatments.

Experiments using naturally fluorescent or radiolabelled compounds have provided significant data on drug uptake and release in individual living cells [28,29] and have demonstrated the crucial role of the membrane in allowing sufficient drug concentration in the cell or not.

On the one hand, it has been shown that cells resistant to methotrexate are not resistant to other structurally different drugs. On the other hand, cell line variants selected by growth in the presence of colchicine also become resistant to other unrelated compounds: vinblastine, vincristine, ectoposide (VP-16), teniposide (VM-26), dactinomycin (actinomycin D), doxorubicin (adriamycin), daunomycin. These cross-reacting agents belong to different families of drugs and are active through different pathways: they interfere with the microtubular organisation, are DNA intercalators or inhibitors of DNA polymerase. They have in common the property of being "natural product" derivatives with a polycyclic structure and are poorly soluble in water. Acquired resistance to these agents is called multiple drug-resistance (mdr).

A series of experiments has demonstrated that the presence of mdr is associated with selective changes in membrane permeability [28-30] leading to altered drug uptake and release in individual living cells. It has been found that the binding of cytotoxic agents to membrane vesicles is enhanced in resistant cells [31] and associated with a low intracellular level.

The binding sites are located on a membrane protein with a molecular weight of 150-180 kD (P-glycoprotein) [32]. The molecular weight, the glycoprotein structure and immunological properties are very similar among cells from different species (hamster, mouse, human). The same membrane protein is associated with resistance to drugs acting on different intracellular target sites as indicated above [23]. Its homology with a bacterial transport protein has led to an explicative model for multiple drug resistance [34]. Both possess an extensive transmembrane region resembling those found in poreforming membrane proteins and involved in bacterial transport protein.

Recent experiments also support evidence that the expression of this P-glycoprotein is responsible for a rapid efflux resulting in low drug concentration in resistant cells [28,29]. The amount of protein is correlated with the degree of drug resistance [32,35]. Its overproduction in resistant cells is mediated by gene amplification [36]. Transfection of a full-length cDNA clone from mdr cells confers multidrug resistance on drug sensitive cells [37,38]. The gene amplification could take place after an enhanced expression of the gene [39].

The process of drug-resistance acquisition in cell lines can be partially reversed if the cells are returned to non-selective medium for successive subcultures [40]. Decrease of resistance parallels a reduction in the number of gene copies and a lesser expression of mRNA. However, this reduction is incomplete and heterogeneous in the cell population. Several experiments have shown that resistant cell lines develop a more differentiated morphology and partially lose their tumourigenicity when injected into nude mice [41]. However, these data have not been confirmed in leukaemia cell lines of human origin [42].

The majority of these data have been obtained from experiments on cell lines derived from humans or rodents. Human normal or tumour samples have been analysed more recently, either for their DNA sequences and mRNA expression or for their content in the encoded mdr protein.

It has been found that the distribution of the P glycoprotein and the expression of the corresponding gene is not homogeneous in the body. The highest level of mdr expression is observed in the adrenal, more in the medulla than in the cortex [43,44]. The rise of P glycoprotein expression might be related to the maturation of this organ. It is expressed also in the placenta [45].

The expression of mdr is also elevated in lung, liver, pancreas, and the digestive mucosa. It must be remarked that tumours of these sites usually display a low sensitivity to cytotoxics while tumours like adenocarcinoma of the breast are initially sensitive. These findings support the hypothesis that in physiological conditions, this protein may have a function in the normal secretion of metabolites and various toxic drugs into bile, urine and digestive lumen, and provide protection from various toxic agents ingested in the diet [46].

In addition, it is to be noted that cells experimentally submitted to polycyclic carcinogens develop similar processes of gene amplification [5,47]. As an example, overexpression of P-glycoprotein is associated with the liver response to carcinogens. [48-50]. It has been suggested that carcinogenesis is the result of the selection of one clone which is altered and resistant. This would provide an explanation for tumours which have been induced by chemicals and express a resistant phenotype, and for all kinds of previously untreated tumours which are initially resistant. The process of gene amplification leading to resistance might be facilitated by the genetic instability of transformed cells [6,51].

Other membrane proteins have been found to be associated with the acquired resistance of individual cell lines [52]. Their activity seems to be related also to a mechanism of drug extrusion from resistant cells and a phosphorylation process is required for their activity. Their molecular weight is close to that of mdr: 150, 180 and 210 kDa. In the human genome, another P glycoprotein has been identified [53]. The corresponding cDNA is distinct from mdr, and would appear to correspond to one of the P glycoproteins identifed in the hamster. A new type of resistance to mitoxanthrone, not reversed by verapamil and not correlated with overexpression of the P glycoprotein has recently been identified. It could be related to a novel drug-resistant gene [54].

It can be speculated that these alternative expressions of membrane protein provide an explanation for the variation in cross-resistance and apparent discrepancies between one given protein overexpression and resistance.

In situ hybridisation studies have demonstrated that the human P-glycoprotein sequence is located on chromosome 7q 21 in normal lymphocytes [55] and in resistant cells [56]. In a MCF.7 adriamycin variant, this gene is amplified 60-fold and the corresponding mRNA overexpressed 45-fold. In other resistant cell lines (colon adenocarcinoma and fibrosarcoma), alterations have been identified more frequently on chromosomes 1, 5, 7 and 11, the 7q being the most frequent site of change [57].

Besides the overexpression of the P glycoprotein in the plasma membrane, a low molecular weight cytoplasmic protein (MW 19,000-22,000) has also been reported to be overexpressed [58]. It has been characterised as a calcium binding protein [59,60] but its exact role has not been clarified.

Until now, few data obtained from human biopsies have been correlated with the degree of response to the treatment [43], but there is no doubt that the ability to measure the level of mdr RNA in tumours would be useful and could help to detect those tumours likely to fail to respond to a given drug [42,43,61].

Reversal of the resistance in the presence of pharmacological agents provides a better understanding of the mdr P glycoprotein mechanism of action. Indeed, it has been observed that various agents including calcium channel blockers reverse multidrug resistance, presumably by facilitating drug accumulation inside the cell. Among these agents, verapamil, which is a calcium blocker, inhibits the active outward transport of the drug. [29,62].

In the case of resistance to drugs of the vincristine family, reversal of resistance seems to be related to the same mediator as the activity of the cytotoxin itself. Indeed, the vinca alkaloid acts by binding to a membrane acceptor which is closely related to the multidrug P-150-180 glycoprotein [63,64]. Calcium channel blockers bind to the mdr protein with a high affinity and overcome the resistance by this pathway. They are specific competitive inhibitors of the drug on its target site of action [63]. The same acceptor exhibits cross-reactivity with several cytotoxic drugs including vinblastine, actinomycin D, adriamycin or colchicine [63] in spite of their different mechanism of action. In all cases, the resistance to these drugs is closely related to the overproduction of the mdr protein. Calcium channel blockers overcome the resistance but the mechanism of their action is less related to their efficiency as blockers than to their interaction with mdr by another pathway [64].

The ability of the mdr glycoprotein to pump out the drug is associated with its phosphorylation [65,66]. The protein is located in the plasma membrane. It forms several loops which are located inside the membrane for one part, on the internal face of the membrane for another part. The glycosyl radical is on the external face and phosphorylation takes place on two internal sites. It has been shown that the mdr protein might be an ATPase enzyme that is cAMP and kinase A dependent [67]. However, the agents which interact directly with the protein and reverse the acquired drug resistance (verapamil) enhance the ATPase activity [67]. The exact pathway of this mechanism is not clear but one explicative hypothesis suggests that they act as competitive inhibitors.

Another class of agents, active on mdr reversal, have in common the ability to alter the intracellular flux and degradation of biological products. Among them are chloroquine and other substances (trifluoroperazine, clomiphene and related compounds) which affect the distribution of antibiotics in the hydrophobic/hydrophylic cell compartment [68,69]. Some of them display heterogeneous main biological functions: agents like clomiphene and tamoxifen have a hormonal first-line activity mediated by oestrogen receptors. They are also calmodulin antagonists and inhibit Ca++ dependent protein kinases such as calmodulin kinase and protein kinase C [70-72]. It has been suggested that their activity on acquired drug resistance could be mediated by this pathway. This hypothesis is illustrated by the role of protein kinase C activation in the phorbol-induced multidrug resistance [73]. A cytosolic 20 kDa protein which is overexpressed in mdr cell lines is phosphorylated by this process [73]. However, the exact role of these low molecular cytosolic proteins in multidrug resistance is still unknown [67].

Conclusion

The drugs used in cancer therapy belong to various families. All of them are substances which are not normally introduced into the body. They contribute to reduction of cell replication by interacting at different steps with cellular components, in relation to their own properties.

Among tumour tissues, some display a low sensitivity to drugs regardless of any previous treatment, others are initially sensitive but become resistant after treatment. The acquired resistance may be directed toward unrelated drugs.

These observations suggest that the response to one drug is related to its structure and to its site and mechanism of action. However, the cell capacity of response should preexist in the body and be activated only after treatment. Indeed, in relation to their physiological activity some organs normally display detectable levels of these activities which are enhanced in the cases of acquired resistance: the detoxification activity of liver cells by coupling the toxic agent to the glutathione molecule is an example. Another one is the toxic efflux by colonic and renal cells. Such properties represent a benefit for the body when it is accidentally submitted to dangerous substances. But they represent also a potent limit of the effects which can be expected from drugs potentially active against tumour proliferation.

The initial mechanism of drug resistance acquisition is similar for a variety of drugs acting through different pathways. Whether the amount of the drug target is increased or the capacity of drug extension is enhanced, changes in gene activity are involved: the gene encoding for the responsible enzyme or for one given protein becomes overexpressed and/or amplified.

Experimental investigations on the rise of such changes have led to important findings: there are similarities between the cell response to cytotoxic drugs, to carcinogens and to ionising radiations. This is not surprising since all these agents are known as mutagens in precise conditions. The processes of DNA lesions and repair themselves could lead to overexpression of genes and production of more than one copy. These alterations of DNA might be also facilitated by the instability of the genome of tumour cells and the degree of activity of the gene at the time of the lesion.

Certainly more processes of this type and contributing to drug resistance still have to be discovered. In spite of improved knowledge and understanding of the biological activities which impair the efficiency or the treatment, it is still difficult to overcome all these processes. However, it can be expected that such experimental findings and further data obtained from tumour biopsies will lead to 1) a better selection of drugs for a maximum efficiency on each tumour, associated with minimum damage of normal cells; 2) adequate adaptation of the ratio dose/sequence of drug administration, thereby allowing the degree of acquired resistance to be reduced.

REFERENCES

1   Young CW, Schochetman G, Karnofsky DA: Hydroxy urea-induced inhibition of deoxyribonucleotide synthesis: studies in intact cells. Cancer Res 1967 (27):526-534

2   Choy BK, McClarty GA, Chan AK, Thelander L, Wright JA: Molecular mechanisms of drug resistance involving ribonucleotide reductase: hydroxyurea resistance in a series of clonally related mouse cell lines selected in the presence of increasing drug concentrations. Cancer Res 1988 (48):2029-2035

3   McClarty GA, Chan AK, Engstrom Y, Wright JA, Thelander L: Elevated expression of M1 and M2 components and drug-induced post transcriptional modulation of ribonuleotide reductase in a hydroxyurea resistant mouse cell line. Biochemistry 1987 (26):8004-8011

4   Alt FW, Kellems FR, Bertino JR, Schimke RT: Selective multiplication of dihydrofolate reductase gene in methotrexate-resistant variants of cultured murine cells. J Biol Chem 1978 (253):1357-1370

5   Schimke RT: Gene amplification, drug resistance, and cancer. Cancer Res 1984 (44):1735-1742

6   Fox M, Roberts JJ: Drug resistance and DNA repair. Cancer and Metastasis Rev 1987 (6):261-281

7   Heck MMS, Hittelman WN, Earnshaw WC: Differential expression of DNA topoisomerase I and II during the enkariotic cell cycle. Proc Natl Acad Sci (USA) 1988 (85):1086-1090

8   Hsiang YH, Wu HY, Liu LF: proliferation-dependent regulation of topoisomerase II in cultured human cells. Cancer Res 1988 (48):3230-3235

9   Trask DK, Muller: Stabilization of type I topoisomerase-DNA covalent complexes by actinomycin D. Proc Natl Acad Sci (USA) 1988 (85):1417-1421

10 Rowe TC, Chen GL, Hsiang YH, Liu LF: DNA damage by antitumor acridines mediated by mammalian DNA topoisomerase II. Cancer Res 1986 (46):2021-2026

11 Pommier Y, Schwartz RE, Zwelling LA, Kerrigan D, Mattern MR, Charcosset JY, Jacquemin-Sablon A, Kohn KW: Reduced formation of protein associated DNA strand breaks in chinese hamster cells resistant to topoisomerase II action. Cancer Res 1986 (46):611-616

12 Zwelling LA, Estey E, Silberman L, Doyle S, Hittelman W: Effect of cell proliferation and chromatin conformation of intercalator - induced protein associated DNA cleavage in human brain tumor cells and human fibrobalsts. Cancer Res 1987 (47):251-257

13 Bakic M, Chan D, Freireich EJ, Marton LJ, ZwellingLA: Effect of polyamine depletion by Difluoromethylornithine or (2R,5R)-6-heptyne-2,5-diamine on drug induced topoisomerase II-mediated DNA cleavage and cytotoxicity in human and murine leukemia cells. Cancer Res 1987 (47):6437-6443

14 Pommier Y, Kerrigan D, Schwartz RE, Swack JA, McCendy A: Altered DNA topoisomerase II activity in chinese hamster cells resistant to topoisomerase II inhibitors. Cancer Res 1986 (46):3075-3081

15 Pommier Y, Kerrigan D, Covey JM, Kao-Shan CS, Wang-Peng J: Sister chromatide exchanges, chromosomal aberrations and cytotoxicity produced by antitumor topoisomerase II inhibitors in sensitive (DC 3F) and resistant (DC 3F/9-DHE) chinese hamster cells. Cancer Res 1988 (48):512-516

16 Batist G, Tulpule A, Sinha BK, Katki AG, Myers CE, Cowan KH: Over expression of a novel anionic glutathione transferase in multidrug-resistant human breast cancer cells. J Biol Chem 1986 (261):15544-15549

17 Richon VM, Schulte N, Eastman A: Multiple mechanisms of resistance to cis-diamminedichloroplatinum (II) in murine leukemia L1210 cells.Cancer Res 1987 (47):2056-2061

18 Wang AL, Tew KD: Increased glutathione S-transferase acticity in a cell line with acquired resistance to nitrogen mustard. Cancer Treat Rep 1985 (69): 677-682

19 Deffie AM, Alam T, Senevriatne C, Beenken SW, Batra JK, Shea TC, Henner WD, Goldenberg GJ: Multifactorial resistance to adriamycin : relationship of DNA repair, glutathione transferase activity, drug efflux and P-glycoprotein in cloned cell line of adriamycin-sensitive and -resistant P 388 leukemia. Cancer Res 1988 (48):3595-3602

20 Kano T, Sakai M, Muramatsu M: Structure and expression of a human class π glutathione S-transferase messenger RNA. Cancer Res 1987 (47):5626-5630

21 Tatematsu M, Mera Y, Ito N, Satoh K, Sato K: Relative merits of immunohistochemical demonstration of placental A,B and C forms of glutathione S-Transferase and histochemical demonstration of g-glutamyltransferase as marker of altered foci during liver carcinogenesis of rat. Carcinogenesis 1985 (6):1621-1626

22 Dejong JL, Morgenstern R, Jornvall H, Depierre JW, Tu CPD: Gene expression of rat and human microsomal glutathione transferase. J Biol Chem 1988 (263):8430-8436

23 Rushmore TH, Harris L, Nagai M, Sharma RN, Hayes MA, Cameron RG, Murray RK, Farber E: Purification and characterization of P-52 (Glutathione S.Transferase-P or 7-7) from normal liver and putative preneoplastic liver nodules. Cancer Res 1988 (48):2805-2812

24 Kirkpatrick DL: Modification of antitumor disulfide cytotoxicity by glutathione depletion in murine cells. Cancer Res 1987 (47):4391-4395

25 Green JA, Vistica DT, Young RC, Hamilton TL, Rogan AM, Ozols RF:Potentiation of melfalan cytotoxicity in human ovarian cell lines by glutathione depletion. Cancer Res 1984 (44):5427-5431

26 Russo A, Graff W, Friedman N, Mitchell JB: Selective modulation of glutathione levels in human normal versus tumor cells and subsequent differential response to chemotherapy drugs. Cancer Res 1986 (46):2845-2848

27 Kramer RA, Greene K, Ahmad S, Vistica DT: Chemosensitization of L-Phenylalanine mustard by the thiol-modulating agent buthionine-sulfoximine. Cancer Res 1987 (47):1593-1597

28 Willingham MC, Cornwell MM, Cardarelli CO, Gottesman MM, Pastan I: Single cell analysis of daunomycine uptake and efflux in multidrug-

resistant and sensitive KB cells : effects of Verapamil and other drugs.Cancer Res 1986 (46) : 5941-5946

29 Fojo A, Akiyama SI, Gottesman MM, Pastan I: Reduced drug accumulation in multiply drug-resistant human KB carcinoma cell lines. Cancer Res 1985 (45);3002-3007

30 Siegfried JA, Kennedy KA, Sartorelli AC, Tritton TR: The role of membranes in the mechanism of action of the antineoplastic agent adriamycin. J Biol Chem 1983 (10):339-343

31 Cornwell MM, Gottesman MM, Pastan IH: Increased vinblasine binding to membrane vesicles from multidrug resistant KB cells. J Biol Chem 1986 (261):7921-7928

32 Kartner N, Riordan JR, Ling V: Cell surface P-glycoprotein associated with multidrug resistance in mammalian cell lines. Science 1983 (221):1285-1288

33 Shen D, Cardarelli C, Hwang J, Cornwell M, Richert N, Ishii S, Pastan I, Gotteman MM: Multiple drug-resistant human KB carcinoma cells independently selected for high-level resistance to colchicine, adriamycin or vinblastine show changes in expression of specific proteins.J Biol Chem 1986 (261):7762-7770

34 Gerlach JH, Endicott JA, Juranka PF, Henderson G, Sarangi F, Deuchers KL, LingHomology between P-glycoprotein and a baterial hemolysin transport protein suggest a mode for multidrug resistance. Nature 1986 (324):485-489

35 Shen DW, Fojo A, Roninson JB, Chin R, Soffir R, Pastan I, Gottesman MM: Multidrug resistance of DNA-mediated transformants in linked to transfer of the human mdr1 gene. Mol Cell Biol 1986 (6):4039-4034

36 Riordan JR, Deuchars K, Kartner N, Alon N, Trent J, Ling V: Amplification of P-glycoprotein genes in multigrug-resistant mammalian cell lines. Nature 1985 (232):817-81

37 Gros P, Groop J, Roninson L, Varshavsky A, Housman DE: Isolation and characterization of DNA sequences amplified in multidrug resistant hamster cells. Proc Natl Acad Sci (USA) 1986 (83)337-34

38 Sugimoto Y, Tsuruo T: DNA-mediated transfer and cloning of a human multidrug resistant gene of adriamycin-resistant myelogenous leukemia K562. Cancer Res 1987 (47):2620-2625

39 Shen D, Fojo A, Chin JE, Roninson IB, Richert N, Pastan I, Gottesman MM: Human multidrug-resistant cell lines: increased mdr1 expression can precede gene amplification. Science 1986 (232):643-645

40 Shen DW, Pastan I, Gottesman MM : in situ hybridation analysis of acquisition and loss of the human multidrug-resistant gene. Cancer Res 1988 (48):4334-4339

41 Biedler J, Reihm H, Peterson R, Spengler BA: Membrane mediated drug resistance and phenotypic reversion to normal growth behavior chinese hamster cells. J Natl Cancer Inst 1975 (55):671-680

42 Hill AB, Beck WT, Trent JM: Cytogenetic and molecular characterization of tumors in mdr mice derived from a multidrug resistant human leukemia cell line. Cancer Res 1988 (48):393-398

43 Fojo AT, Ueda K, Slamon DJ, Poplack DG, Gottesman MM, Pastan O: Expression of a multidrug resistance gene in human tumors and tissues. Proc Natl Acad Sci (USA) 1987 (84) :265-269

44 Thiebaut F, Tsuruo T, Hamada H, Gottesman MM, Pastan I, Willingham MC: Cellular localization of the multidrug-resistance gene product P-glycoprotein in normal human tissues. Proc Natl Acad Sci (USA) 1987 (84):7735-7738

45 Sugawara I, Kataoka I, Morishita Y, Hamada H, Tsurudo T, Itoyama S, Mori S: Tissue distribution of P-glycoprotein encoded by a multidrug resistant gene as revealed by monoclonal antibody-MRK 16. Cancer Res 1988 (48):1926-1929

46 Klohs WD, Steinkampf RW: Possible link between the intrinsic drug resistance of colon tumors and a detoxification mechanism of intestinal cells. Cancer Res 1988 (48):3025-3030

47 Sager R, Gadi IK, Stephens L, Grabowy CT: Gene amplification: an example of accelerated evolution in tumourigenic cells. Proc Natl Acad Sci (USA) 1985 (82):7015-7019

48 Cowan KH, Batist G, Tulpule A, Sinha BK, Myers CE: Similar biochemical changes associated with multidrug resistance in human breast cancer cells and carcinogen-induced resistance to xenobiotics in rats. Proc Natl Acad Sci (USA)1986   (83):9328-9332

49 Fairchild CR, Ivy SP, Rushmore T, Lee G, Kod P, Goldsmith ME, Myers CE, Farber E, Cowan KH: Carcinogen-induced mdr overexpression is associated with xenobiotic resistance in rat preneoplastic nodules and hepatocellular carcinomas. Proc Natl Acad Sci (USA) 1987 (84):7701-7705

50 Thorgeirsson SS, Huber BE, Sorrell S, Fojo A, Pastan I, Gottesman MM: Expression of the multidrug-resistant gene in hepatocarcinogenesis and regenerating rat liver. Science 1987 (236):1120-1122

51 Cifone MA, Fidler IJ : Increasing metastatic potential is associated with increasing genetic instability of clones isolated from murine neoplasms. Proc Natl Acad Sci (USA) 1981 (78):6949-6952

52 McGrath T, Center MS: Mechanisms of multidrug resistance in HL60 cells : evidence that a surface membrane distinct from P-glycoprotein contributes to reduced cellular accumulation of drug. Cancer Res 1988 (48):3959-3963

53 Van der Blieck AM, Baas F, Ten Houte de Lange T, Kooiman PM, Van der Velde-Koerts T, Borst P; The human mdr 3 genes encodes a novel P-glycoprotein homologue and gives rise to alternatively mRNA in the liver. The Embo Journal 1987 (6):3325-3331

54 Dalton WS, Cress AE, Alberts DS, Trent JM: Cytogenetic and phenotypic analysis of a human colon carcinoma cell line resistant to mitoxantrone. Cancer Res 1988 (48):1882-1888

55 Fairchild CR, Ivy SP, Kad-Shan CS, Whang-Peng J, Rosen N, Israel MA, Melera PW, Cowan KH, Goldsmith ME: Isolation of amplified over expressed DNA sequences from adriamycin-resistant human breast cancer cells. Cancer Res 1987 (47): 5141-5148

56 Fojo A, Lebo R, Shimizu N, Chin JE, Roninson IB, Merlino GT, Gottesman MM, Pastan I: Localization of multidrug resistance-associated DNA sequences

to human chromosome 7. Somatic Cell Mol Genet 1986 (12):415-420

57 Slovak ML, Hoeltge GA, Trent JM: Cytogenetic alterations associated with the acquisition of Doxorubicin resistance : possible significance of chromosomes 7 alterations. Cancer Res 1987 (47):6646-6652

58 Meyers MB, Biedler J: Increased synthesis of low molecular weight protein in vincristine-resistant cells. Biochem Biophys Res Commun 1981 (99):228-235

59 Koch G, Smith M, Twentyman P, Wright K: Identification of a novel calcium-binding protein (CP22) in multidrug-resistant murine and hamster cells. FEBS Lett 1986 (195):275-279

60 Hamada H, Okochi E, Oh-Hara T, Tsuruo T: Purification of the M2 22,000 calcium-binding protein (Sorcin) associated with multidrug resistance and its detection with monoclonal antibodies. Cancer Res 1988 48):3173-3178

61 Fuqua SAW, Moretti-Rojas IM, Schneider SL, McGuire WL: P-glycoprotein expression in human breast cancer cells. Cancer Res 1987 (47):2103-210

62 Tsuruo T, Iida H, Tsukagoshi S, Sakurai Y: Overcoming of vincristine resistance in P 388 leukemia in vivo in vitro through enhanced cytotoxicity of vincristine and vinblastine by verapamil. Cancer Res 1981(41):1967-1972

63 Safa AR, Glover CJ, Sewell JL, Meyers MB, Biedler JL, Felsted RL: Identification of the multidrug resistance-related membrane glycoprotein as an acceptor for calcium channel blockers. J. Biol Chem 1987 (262):7884-7888

64 Cornwell MM, Pastan I, Gottesman MM: Certain calcium channel blockers bind specifically to multidrug human KB carcinoma membrane vesicles and inhibit drug binding to P-glycoprotein. J Biol Chem 1987 (262):2166-2170

65 Mellado W, Horwitz SB: Phosphorylation of the multidrug resistance associated glycoprotein. Biochem 1987 (26):6900-6904

66 Hamada H, Hagiwara K, Nakajima T, Tsuruo T: Phosphorylation of the M2 170,000 to 180,000 glycoprotein specific of verapamil, trifluoroperazine and phorbol esters. Cancer Res 1987 (47):2860-2868

67 Hamada H, Tsuruo T: Characterization of the ATPase activity of the M2 170,000 to 180,000 membrane glycoprotein (P-glycoprotein) associated with multidrug resistance in K562/ADM cells. Cancer Res 1988 (48):4926-4932

68 Ramu A, Glaubiger D, Fuks Z: Reversal of acquired resistance to doxorubicin in P 388 murine leukemia cells by tamoxifen and other triparanol analogs. Cancer Res 1984 (44):4392-4395

69 Hindenburg A, Baker MA, Gleyzer E, Stewart VJ, Case N, Taub RN: Effect of verapamil and other agents on the distribution of anthracyclines and on reversal of drug resistance. Cancer Res 1987 (47):1421-1425

70 Tsuruo T, Iida H, Tsukagoshi S, Sakenai Y: Potentiation of vincristine and adriamycin effects in human hemopoietic tumor cell lines by calcium antagonists and calmodulin inhibitors. Cancer Res 1983 (43): 2267-2272

71 Tsuruo T, Iida H, Nojiri M, Tsukagoshi S, Sakurai Y: Circumvention of vincristine and adriamycin resistance in vitro and in vivo by calcium influx blockers. Cancer Res 1983 (43):2905-2910

72 Ganapathi R, Grabowski D: Enhancement of sensitivity of adriamycin in resistant P 388 leukemia by the calmodulin inhibitor trifluoroperazine.Cancer Res 1983 (43):3636-363

73 Fine RL, Patel J, Chabner BA: Phorbol esters induce multidrug Resistance in human breast cancer cells. Proc Natl Acad Sci (USA) 1988 (85):582-586

Integration of Quality-of-Life Issues into Clinical Trials of Breast Cancer

R.D. Gelber[1], A. Goldhirsch[2], R.J. Simes[3], P. Glasziou[3] and M. Castiglione[4]

1 Harvard School of Public Health and Dana-Farber Cancer Institute, Boston MA, U.S.A.
2 Division of Oncology, Ospedale San Giovanni, Bellinzona, and Ospedale Civico, Lugano, Switzerland
3 Ludwig Institute for Cancer Research, Sydney, Australia
4 International Breast Cancer Study Group, Bern, Switzerland

Summary

The medical community has accepted randomised trials with mixed feelings. Most physicians do not enter their patients in such trials, primarily because relying on a random chance mechanism is not considered an acceptable way of choosing therapy. For trials concerning adjuvant systemic therapy for breast cancer, the typical reduction of early mortality for treated patients is small. Randomised trials would no longer be needed if a therapeutic breakthrough representing a large improvement in overall survival were available.

In reality, the 75-85% of patients who die of the disease despite treatment represent the potential for improvement in the therapy of the disease. Because the impact of treatment on relapse rates appears earlier than survival effects in all adjuvant therapy trials, and because the value of time without relapse in terms of the quality of life of the patients is as yet poorly defined, we have generalised our method of comparing treatment attitudes to include individual qualitative judgment values. The generalisation includes: 1) a comparison of two populations based upon an overall value given to each period of life either with or without breast cancer related events; 2) the prospective evaluation by each patient of her perception of the quality of her life during each time period (i.e., with toxic effects of drugs, of living without and with relapse); 3) integration of individual patient perceptions regarding the value of time spent with toxicity today as opposed to an uncertain outcome for the future. The experience gained from integrating quality-of-life issues into clinical trials for breast cancer might also be applied to other diseases characterised by a chronic course, toxic treatments and gains in periods of relative or absolute freedom from toxic effects or progressive disease.

Introduction

Most patients with operable breast cancer relapse and die of the disease. The annual relapse rate is relatively low and is related to prognostic variables. Even for patients with metastases in axillary nodes the annual relapse rate is about 10% per year. The annual mortality rate for this population is about 5% per year [1]. Improvements in outcome include a significant reduction of relapses seen in most of the individual trials investigating adjuvant systemic therapies [2] and a 15-25% reduction in the odds of death within 5 years. An overview combining data from all available relevant randomised trials was required to demonstrate the presence of these treatment effects statistically [3]. The considerable efforts being made presently to improve these results include investigation of the ideal timing for administration of adjuvant therapy, evaluation of intensive treatment regimens which require autologous bone marrow transplantation, use of recombinant colony-stimulating factors to reduce bone marrow toxicity, and study of hormonal agents used in association with chemotherapy. It is unlikely, however, that a definitive breakthrough will be achieved by these approaches and it might be anticipated that advances in the treatment of operable breast cancer in terms of overall survival improvement will continue to be of small magnitude.

Such a prospect underscores the need for alternative evaluation methods which take into account the well-being of the patients. The following facts might be considered:
1. There is an increased tendency to treat patients with node-negative disease [4] whose risk for relapse is smaller than that of women with node-positive disease (for whom the value of systemic adjuvant therapy has been established during the past 2 decades).
2. Many physicians are more aware of issues of quality of life. An increasing number of health care professionals understand that the simplistic approach to cancer treatment, "better to live more decently even if for a shorter period," represents a logical error: "shorter" in most cases is related to "worse" in advanced disease [5] and probably also in the adjuvant setting [6].
3. Adapting treatment results from clinical trials to the individual patient situation is very difficult and requires certain assumptions, a number of which are derived empirically. This of course is acceptable since many aspects of modern medicine relate to empirical experience. It can very easily become a matter of controversy, however, especially if the treatment results in terms of disease control are of modest magnitude and borderline significance, while the side effects and costs of treatment are acute and obvious.

Additional endpoints which take into account factors related to the well-being of the patients represent an obviously important tool for decision-making when the treatment-choice situation is such as that currently applying for operable breast cancer.

Development of Comparison Methods

The TWiST Methodology

In the E.S.O. Monograph, Endocrine Therapy of Breast Cancer II [7], we described the TWiST methodology which was applied to a data set including 463 postmenopausal patients with N+ breast cancer who were randomised into Ludwig Study III to receive either a chemoendocrine therapy (cyclophosphamide, methotrexate, 5-fluorouracil, prednisone and tamoxifen = CMFp+T) for one year *or* endocrine therapy alone (p+T) for one year *or* no adjuvant therapy (Observation). The Time Without Symptoms of disease and Toxic effects of treatment was considered as the endpoint. TWiST was calculated by subtracting from overall survival all time periods for which some subjective toxicity was noted, and all time following symptomatic systemic relapse that involved additional treatment intervention. This pragmatic approach has been the basis for the development of the methodology, but could hardly be considered a reliable way to evaluate the actual impact of treatment felt by the patients. Subjective toxicity and symptoms of relapse are obviously far from being pleasant conditions of life, but most women with breast cancer will nevertheless consider any time periods to have some value greater than death [8].

Q-TWiST Methodology

In order to allocate some value greater than zero to time periods during which the patient is alive with or without the occurrence of a quality-of-life-related event, the following definitions were established (using the same criteria as for the TWiST method):
a) the time period during the course of follow-up when an individual patient experiences *subjective toxic effects* (TOX),
b) time following systemic relapse (REL),
c) time spent recovering from treatment of isolated *local recurrence* (LC), and
d) any remaining survival time left after subtracting a), b) and c) which represents *time without symptoms and toxicity* (TWiST).

For reasons of convenience, in the subsequent discussion LR will be incorporated within REL.

Quality-adjusted survival analysis is performed by considering utility coefficients u_t and u_r, taking values between 0 and 1, to represent the value relative to TWiST, of toxic periods (TOX) and time after relapse (REL),

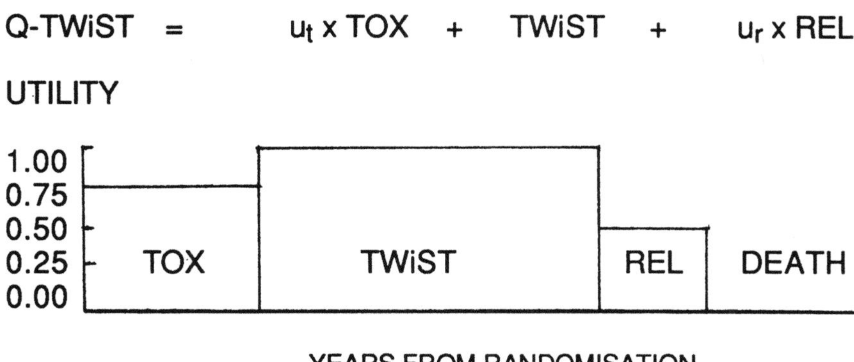

Fig. 1. Calculation of Q-TWiST: weighted summation of time periods TOX, TWiST and REL. Utility coefficients of ut=0.75 for TOX and ur=0.50 for REL are illustrated

respectively. Quality-adjusted survival relative to TWiST (Q-TWiST) for a patient who experiences an overall survival composed of TOX, TWiST and REL is calculated as:

$$Q\text{-}TWiST = u_t \times TOX + TWiST + u_r \times REL$$

Figure 1 illustrates the way in which u_t and u_r influence the addition of time periods to the "baseline" TWiST for arbitrarily chosen values of 0.75 for u_t and 0.50 for u_r.

Population estimates of Q-TWiST achieved for a specific treatment regimen are obtained by partitioning overall survival up to a specified time from randomisation into 3 regions (see Figures 2A, 2B and 2C). The regions are distinguished by curves for duration of toxic effects, time to systemic relapse, and overall survival time. The average amounts of time spent in TOX, TWiST and REL for each treatment group up to a specified cutoff time from randomisation are estimated by the areas between the curves as shown. These averages are then combined as a weighted sum according to the above equation to obtain an average Q-TWiST for each treatment.

Treatments are compared using a spectrum of u_t and u_r values, and threshold values of u_t and u_r are determined in greater detail in a recent publication [9]. Figure 3 shows the

threshold analysis for Ludwig Study III with cutoff at 7 years from randomisation. The bold lines divide the figures into 3 regions where each treatment is favoured according to the values placed on time with toxicity (u_t) and time following systemic relapse (u_r) relative to TWiST. The dashed lines show the thresholds between pairs of treatments.

Table 1. Components of Q-TWiST for treatments evaluated in Ludwig Trial III. Average months of TOX, TWiST and REL accumulated within 7 years of randomisation, with Q-TWiST calculated for arbitrary utility coefficients ($u_t = u_r = 0.5$). (Standard errors are shown in parentheses)

	CMFp+T	p+T	Observation
TOX	9.6 (0.4)	2.0 (0.3)	0.0 (0.0)
TWiST	50.3 (2.5)	47.1 (2.7)	41.5 (2.6)
REL	7.1 (1.1)	12.9 (1.4)	20.9 (1.8)
Q-TWiST ($u_t = u_r = 0.5$)	58.7 (1.1)	54.6 (2.3)	51.9 (2.2)

CMFp+T	= cyclophosphamide, methotrexate, 5-fluorouracil, prednisone + tamoxifen (chemoendocrine therapy)
p+T	= prednisone + tamoxifen (endocrine therapy alone)
Observation	= no adjuvant therapy

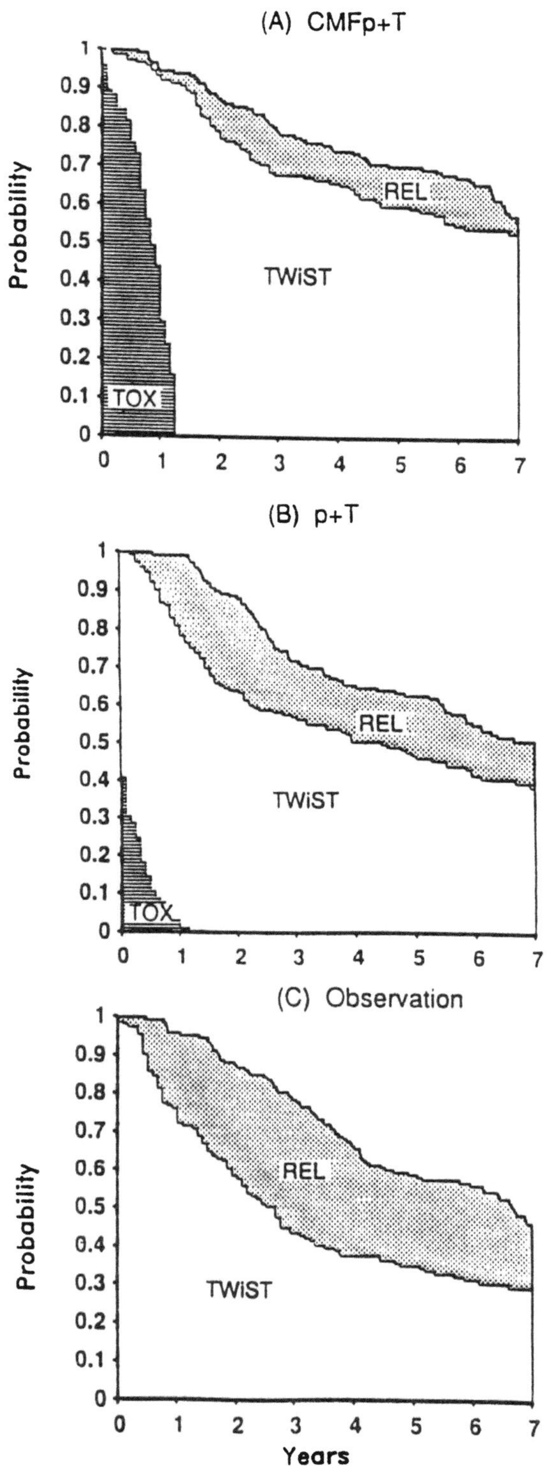

Fig. 2. Time accumulated up to 7 years from randomisation is partitioned for each treatment group by curves for time with toxicity, time to systemic relapse, and overall survival. Areas between these curves yield population average values for TOX, TWiST, and REL. Panel A = CMFp+T, panel B = p+T, and panel C = Observation.

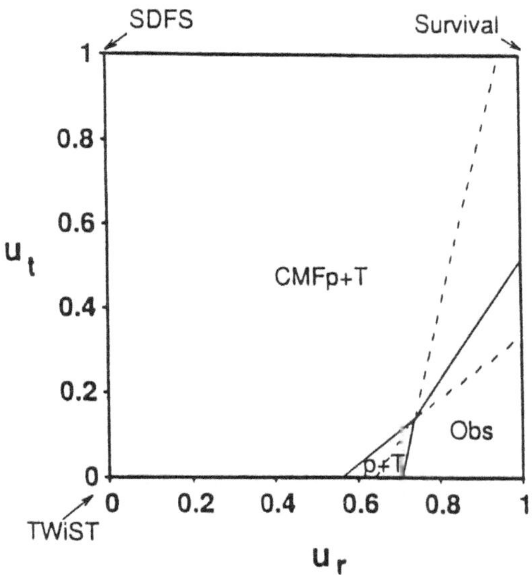

Fig. 3. Threshold analysis for Ludwig Trial III comparing average Q-TWiST values accumulated after 7 years from randomisation. Lines are drawn for values u_t and u_r which yield equal values of average Q-TWiST between treatment pairs

The average times accumulated in TOX, TWiST and REL during 7 years which are graphically present in Figure 2 may also be described numerically. These average values are summarised in Table 1. The calculation of Q-TWiST is illustrated by a weighted combination of these components using $u_t=u_r=0.50$. Based on these arbitrary values for the utility coefficients the average Q-TWiST accumulated during 7 years (84 maximum possible months) for chemoendocrine therapy was 58.7 months - 4.1 months longer than for endocrine therapy alone ($p=0.20$), and 6.7 months longer than for the observation group ($p=0.05$). The threshold analysis (Fig. 3) shows that CMFp+T is the preferred treatment for a wide range of plausible values of ut and ur. For the specific values at the corners of Figure 3 treatment comparisons are for systemic-disease-free survival ($u_t=1$, $u_r=0$), TWiST ($u_t=0$, $u_r=0$) and overall survival ($u_t=1$, $u_r=1$). It is important to note that these thresholds are based upon 7-year figures, and further follow-up will enhance any advantage of CMFp+T over p+T or Observation, moving the thresholds further toward the lower right-hand corner.

In order to provide some data about the statistical uncertainty of the results we display the threshold lines together with their

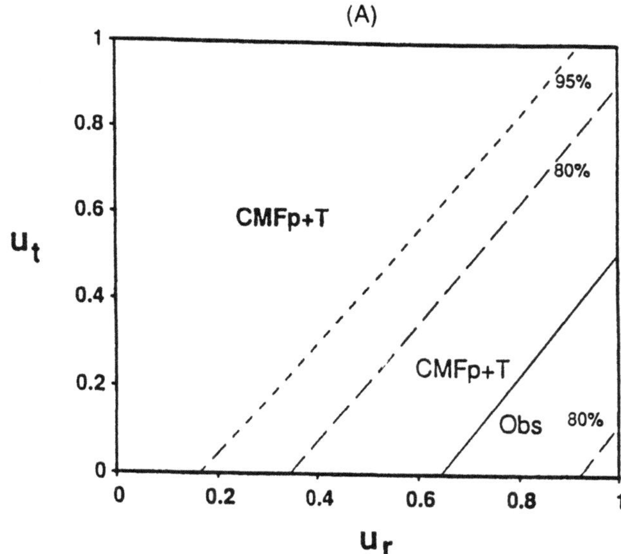

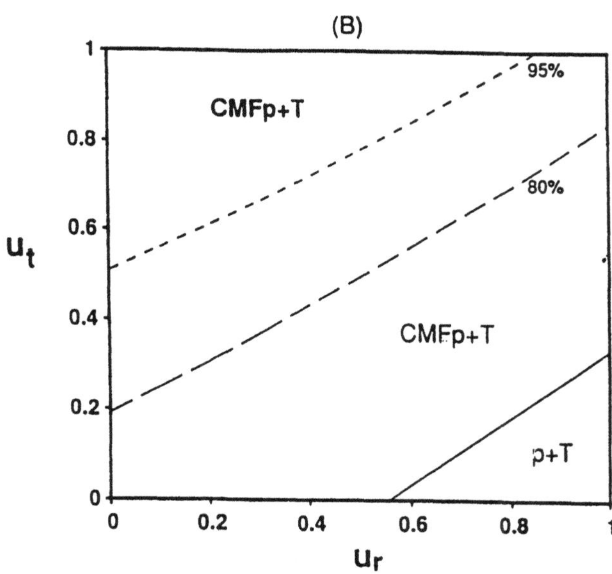

Fig. 4. Pairwise treatment comparisons for (A) CMFp+T versus Observation and (B) CMFp+T versus p+T showing 80% and 95% confidence regions

confidence intervals. The comparisons of CMFp+T vs. Observation (Fig. 4A) and CMFp+T vs. p+T (Fig. 4B) are described. For the first comparison there is a statistically significant difference in favour of CMFp+T for most values of u_t and u_r. The confidence regions for CMFp+T vs. p+T are still wide and the range of values of u_t and u_r for which the chemoendocrine therapy is statistically significantly preferred is small.

Our example is based upon the trial results at 7 years of median follow-up time. The chemoendocrine therapy involves early toxicity but later gains which exceed those of the endocrine therapy alone. The evolution of the differences in average Q-TWiST (for $u_t=u_r=0.5$) between treated and control groups is displayed in Figure 5A. As time from randomisation increases, the early losses due to toxic effects are counterbalanced by the gains associated with delayed relapse, so that an average overall gain for the population of treated patients begins to emerge at 3 to 4 years after operation. The evolution of results for other endpoints of TWiST (Fig. 5B) and overall survival (Fig. 5C) can be displayed in a similar fashion. This practice of displaying the results in terms of different endpoints illustrates the clinical utility of the methods, since the dimension of time from diagnosis (or from primary treatment) is added for comparison with the conventional assessments of disease-free survival and overall survival.

Adding Other Arbitrary Utility Coefficients to Q-TWiST

Some other ideas related to economical sciences may be borrowed for our attempt to integrate quality-of-life-oriented values to the analysis of breast cancer therapies. One year commencing from the present time might have intrinsically more value than one year commencing from some time (5 years, say) in the future. A discount rate per year of life without relapse may be considered to express the fact that the loss of present time due to immediate toxicity might be too high a price for gaining an equal amount of time in the future. Similarly, delaying a relapse that would have occurred late might not be as valuable as delaying an early recurrence. A delayed relapse also has a better prognosis [10] in terms of survival, and therefore some kind of discount might be justified.

Criticism may obviously be raised against this discounting policy due to the fact that many patients might reason according to the "insurance mentality" - an investment today (in terms of toxic effects to all) for a chance of reduction of odds of relapse in the future should not be penalised regardless of when the relapse eventually occurs. It is important to

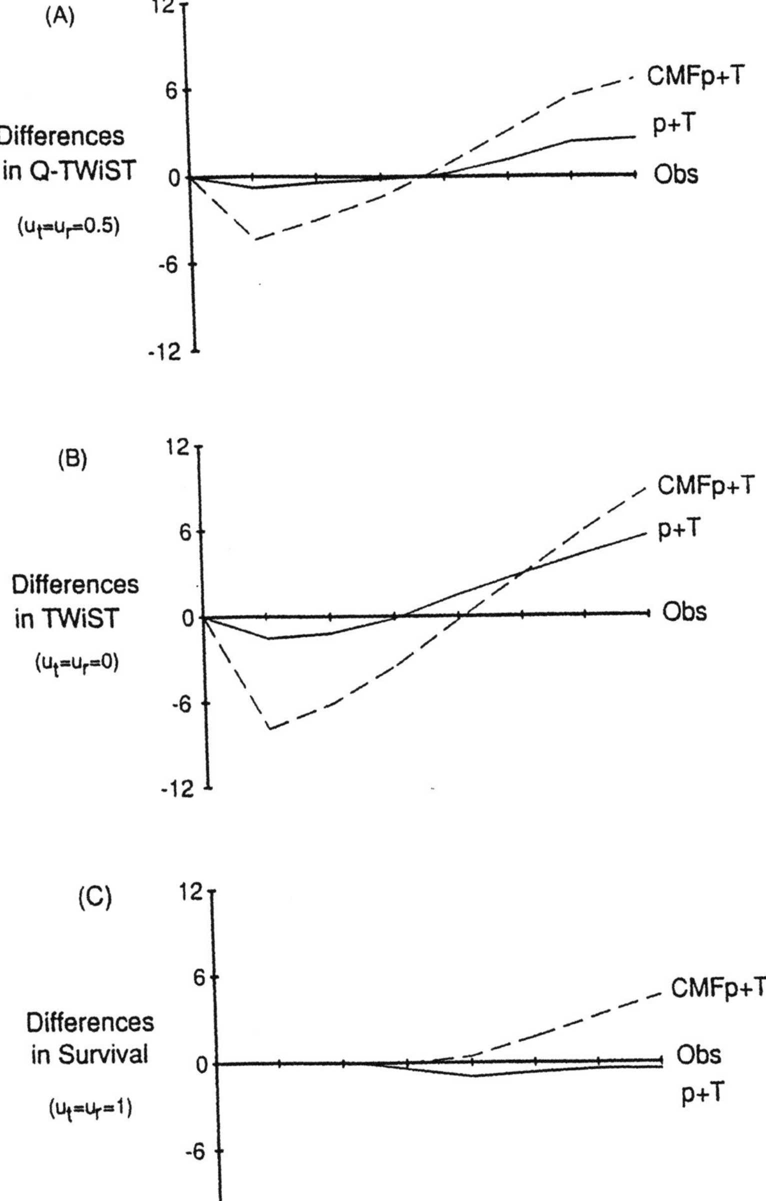

Fig. 5. Treatment differences relative to Observation as functions of time from randomisation. Differences are in terms of average months of Q-TWiST accumulated since randomisation for:
(A) Q-TWiST with arbitrary values ut=ur=0.5
(B) TWiST (i.e., Q-TWiST with ut=ur=0)
(C) Overall survival (i.e., Q-TWiST with ur=ut=1)

evaluate the prospective perception of the patient regarding a delayed relapse, whether early or late. The effects of the discounting of time by 10% per year on our results within 7 years is displayed in the threshold analysis presented in Figure 6. In spite of the lower value of late accruing gains, chemoendocrine therapy is still preferred for the majority of utility coefficients.

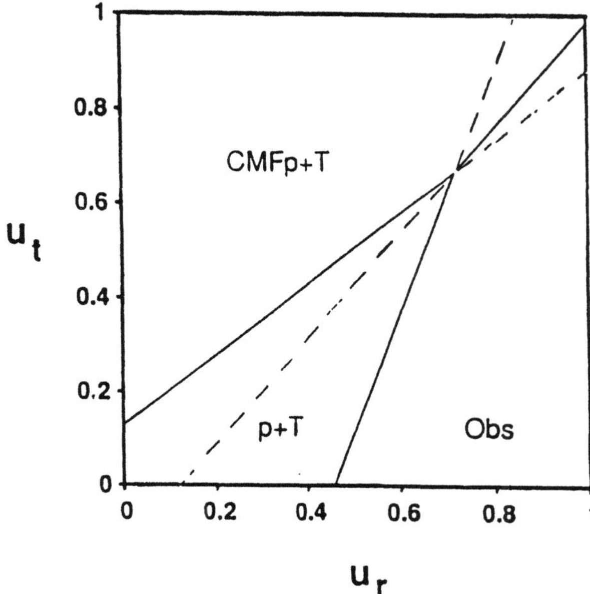

Fig. 6. Threshold analysis for Ludwig Trial III within 7 years from randomisation with the value of future time discounted at 10% per year

But What Is THE SINGLE Answer Provided by a Q-TWiST Analysis?

Four values must be specified in order to obtain a unique solution for average Q-TWiST treatment comparisons derived from a clinical trial dataset: the two utility coefficients u_t and u_r, the time from diagnosis considered for the comparison, and the discount factor. Some might be uncomfortable with the prospect that a clinical trial will not yield a definitive answer recommending a treatment for application to all patients. Yet, quality of life is a philosophical issue which in fact cannot have such a unique answer. The Q-TWiST methodology is developed with this spirit, recognising that choices are required to be individualised, and establishing a framework within which the parameters for treatment choice can be explicitly introduced.

Specifically, consider the choice of u_t and u_r, the utility coefficients associated with times in toxicity and times after relapse. Using the threshold analyses displayed in Figure 3, one can determine the values of u_t and u_r for which the chemoendocrine therapy is preferred to either of the other two treatment op

tions. If, based on subjective feelings, toxic effects are not considered to be too debilitating compared with the impact on quality of life of a systemic relapse, then u_t is higher than u_r and the data favour chemoendocrine therapy. This is the "insurance mentality" which makes some prospective payment socially acceptable in order for the possibility to be covered for some future calamity. Note that the subjective feelings of relative worth might be derived from the physician (motivated by a prejudice to treat or not to treat), by the patient (who clearly expresses a preference relating to her personal life status at the time), or by the physician using clues and impressions derived from feelings expressed by the patient.

In fact, given that a particular treatment choice is made (e.g. use chemoendocrine therapy rather than no adjuvant treatment), the threshold analysis in Figure 3 defines the implicit relative values of u_t and u_r that apply. In this way the prejudices of physicians who choose a particular treatment strategy are described in terms of how they must weigh the relative value of the time periods TOX, TWiST and REL.

The other two variables (time from diagnosis and discount rate) are easier to handle. The time from diagnosis is constrained by the maturity of the dataset. In order to consider results which are less subject to statistical fluctuations, we generally extrapolate no further than the median follow-up of the study cohort. The choice of discount factor is related to the patient's age, family situation at the time of diagnosis, and the relative value of the next year as compared with a year several years to the future. A time trade-off methodology might be useful for determining the discount rate. The exact specification of the discount rate is, however, not crucial for the application of the methodology, because even with a discount of 10% per year (about 40% over a cumulative 5-year period) conclusions are not much altered from a zero discount analysis.

The importance of the analysis is to recognise its subjective nature and explicitly define the parameters that impact upon treatment choice. Integrating individual patient perceptions into the analysis of treatment choice is the next logical step to increase the clinical application of the methodologic framework.

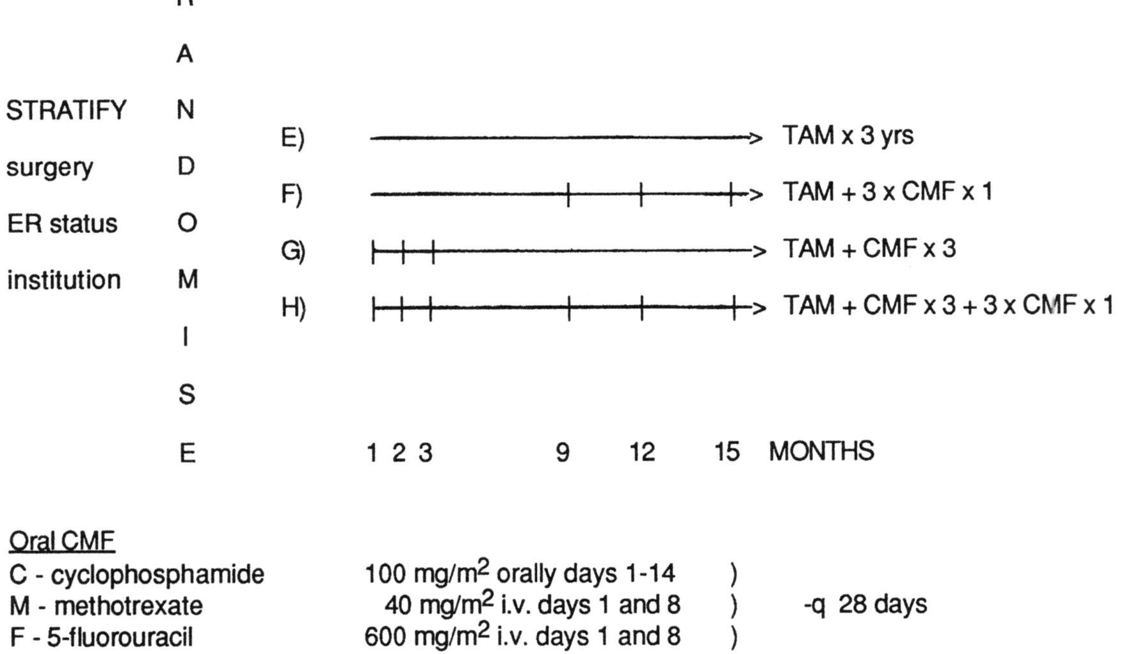

Oral CMF
C - cyclophosphamide   100 mg/m^2 orally days 1-14   )
M - methotrexate   40 mg/m^2 i.v. days 1 and 8   )   -q 28 days
F - 5-fluorouracil   600 mg/m^2 i.v. days 1 and 8   )

TAM = tamoxifen 20 mg daily for 3+ years

Fig. 7. Designs for International Breast Cancer Study Group (IBCSG) Trials VI and VII: Adjuvant therapy for women
with operable node-positive breast cancer

Integrating Perceptions and Opinions of Individual Patients into the Analysis of Treatment Results

The development of the TWiST and Q-TWiST methodologies was based upon the perception and biases of physicians as to the values of life periods. The direct possibility to integrate the patients' own value judgments into the analysis was not possible because of the lack of prospectively collected information. The idea, however, has matured rather early during the developmental process and some instruments are being used in recent trials of systemic adjuvant therapy. The objective is to assess patient coping, well-being and subjective burden of some toxicities to obtain relative values for TOX, TWiST and REL directly from the population of study patients. The trials in which these instruments are being tested are outlined in Figure 7 [11].

Some initial cycles of chemotherapy may be administered with reintroduction of 3 single cycles (days 1 through 14) delivered at 3-monthly intervals later in the patient follow-up (e.g. months 9, 12 and 15).

The patients are questioned every 3 months concerning their well-being and the extent of disturbance caused by treatment. These are compared to a baseline evaluation obtained before the start of any adjuvant systemic treatment. Patients are requested to give the same information one month after the first relapse. Linear Analogue Self Assessments (LASA [8]) provide patient perceptions of adjustment/coping, physical well-being, mood, and appetite. A self-administered adjective checklist is also used to evaluate general well-being at each assessment. These data will help to define values of u_t and u_r that apply to a population of breast cancer patients.

REFERENCES

1   Nemoto T, Vana J, Bedwani RN et al: Management and survival of female breast cancer. Results of a national survey by the American College of Surgeons. Cancer 1980 (45):2917-2924
2   Henderson IC: Adjuvant systemic treatment for early breast cancer. Current Problems in Cancer 1987 (II):125-207
3   UK-BCTSC/UICC/WHO. Review of mortality results in randomised trials in early breast cancer. Lancet 1984 (i):1205
4   Goldhirsch A, Gelber RD: Adjuvant systemic therapy for breast cancer patients without lymph node metastases (N-). European School of Oncology Monographs (this volume)
5   Coates A, Gebski V, Bishop JF et al for the Australian-New Zealand Breast Cancer Trials Group, Clinical Oncological Society of Australia. Improving the quality of life during chemotherapy for advanced breast cancer: a comparison of intermittent and continuous treatment strategies. N Engl J Med 1987 (317):1490-1495
6   Gelber RD, Goldhirsch A, Castiglione M, Price K, Isley M, Coates A, for the Ludwig Breast Cancer Study Group. Time without symptoms and toxicity (TWiST): A quality-of-life-oriented endpoint to evaluate adjuvant therapy. In: Salmon SE (ed) Adjuvant Therapy of Cancer V. Grune & Stratton, Orlando 1987 pp 455-465
7   Gelber RD, Goldhirsch A: Evaluating the benefits of therapies for breast cancer. In: Cavalli F (ed) Endocrine Therapy of Breast Cancer II. ESO Monographs, Springer Verlag, Berlin 1987 pp 21-32
8   Coates A, Fischer Dillenbeck C, McNeal DR et al: On the receiving end - II. Linear analogue self-assessment (LASA) in evaluation of the quality of life of cancer patients receiving therapy. Eur J Cancer Clin Oncol 1983 (19):1633-1637
9   Goldhirsch A, Gelber RD, Simes RJ, Glasziou P, Coates A: Costs and benefits of adjuvant therapy in breast cancer. A quality adjusted survival analysis. J Clin Oncol (in press)
10 Goldhirsch A, Gelber RD, Castiglione M: Relapse of breast cancer after adjuvant treatment in premenopausal and perimenopausal women: patterns and prognoses. J Clin Oncol 1988 (6):89-97
11 Goldhirsch A, Gelber RD, for the Ludwig Breast Cancer Study Group. Adjuvant therapy for breast cancer: The Ludwig Breast Cancer Trials 1987. In: Salmon SE (ed) Adjuvant Therapy of Cancer V. Grune & Stratton, Orlando 1987 pp 297-309

Adjuvant Systemic Therapy for Breast Cancer Patients Without Lymph Node Metastases (N-)

A. Goldhirsch [1] and R.D. Gelber [2]

1) Division of Oncology, Ospedale San Giovanni, Bellinzona and Ospedale Civico, Lugano, Switzerland
2) Harvard School of Public Health and Dana-Farber Cancer Institute, Boston, MA, U.S.A.

Summary

Several issues have recently been raised with respect to the treatment of patients diagnosed as having no axillary metastases after removal of breast cancer and axillary clearance. Patients with N- disease who were treated in the more recent controlled clinical trials have higher relapse rates than those entered in the earlier series from which our perception of prognosis for these patients has been derived. This could be due to a reporting bias, to a selection of patients for study who have a worse prognosis, or because the prognosis for N- breast cancer patients in general has in fact changed from what it was a decade or so ago.

A second important issue is the fact that major trials using either systemic endocrine therapy or chemotherapy have yielded significant improvement in terms of disease-free survival. Adjuvant therapy policies - particularly those affecting women who elect not to be treated within the framework of a clinical trial - are once again in a state of re-evaluation. This summary makes the point that women with N- breast cancer should be treated within clinical trials because the many factors which must be considered for therapy decision-making can most efficaciously be assessed within such a framework.

Introduction

Approximately 40-60% of the patients who are diagnosed as having breast cancer have no metastases in their axillary lymph nodes [1]. The information about the prognosis of these patients is based upon observations made one or more decades ago. If breast cancer is now being diagnosed earlier, the chances are that the majority of the patients will have no detectable disease in their axillary nodes. In fact, the proportion of patients who are being diagnosed with earlier stage of disease is increasing. Screening programmes have been shown to be effective for reducing mortality. However, applying previously reported stage-specific mortality rates to the shifted distribution of breast cancers by stage diagnosed today would suggest an even greater mortality reduction than that observed [2]. This is especially true for younger women (<55 years old) for whom mortality reduction from screening has been marginal in spite of increased detection of node-negative disease. An explanation is that the increased percentage of patients with node-negative disease have tumours which are more aggressive, and therefore would have appeared initially as node-positive disease during the era prior to the introduction of screening programmes and community education. The diagnosis of node-negative breast cancer no longer represents the universally favourable prognosis that it once did.

In Ludwig V, a trial conducted from 1981 to 1985, 2504 patients were accrued *before* the axillary spread of the disease was known

38 A. Goldhirsch and R.D. Gelber

(due to perioperative randomisation). Fifty-one per cent of the women were found to have no metastases in their axillary nodes [3]. In countries with ongoing screening programmes (e.g. Sweden), the prevalence of N- breast cancer has reached 70%. Some selected patients have entered trials designed to investigate the effectiveness of systemic adjuvant therapy, and early results have recently been released. This chapter analyses the evidence available concerning adjuvant therapy in patients with N- breast cancer.

Prognosis of N- Breast Cancer

The use of adjuvant therapy is related to a variety of factors, including:
i) The prognosis of the population at risk.
ii) The definition of a subpopulation at high risk of relapse (to which the knowledge concerning treatment effects accumulated from N+ breast cancer may be applied).
iii) The definition of a population at low risk of relapse for which adjuvant therapy would clearly be over-treatment.
iv) The identification of prognostic factors which are applicable to N- breast cancer *today*.

Table 1 summarises, in terms of relapse-free and survival percentages, the prognosis of patients with N- disease who were included in selected series in which no question of systemic adjuvant therapy was posed. Only the most recent series (NSABP Trial B-06) includes patients with relapse rates exceeding 25% within 5 years.

Over the years various factors have been investigated in the effort to establish a prognostic value in N- breast cancer patients. It has become clear from trials which accrued both N+ and N- patients that the relative impact of adjuvant systemic therapy on outcome is likely to be similar in the two populations. The question of whether or not to administer adjuvant therapy to patients classified as N- is directly related to the risk of recurrence and death. The following prognostic factors were

Table 1. Outcome following local treatment alone for patients with N- breast cancer in selected series

Study	Relapse-free % at 5 years	Survival % at 5 years
Milan, 1st series [4]	79%	88%
Milan, subsequent series [5]	76%	88%
Milan T$_1$ trials [6]	90%	92%
NSABP B-01 [7]	82%	78%
NSABP B-04 [8]	85%	83%
NSABP B-06 [9]	77%-67%*	88%-87%*

* in the different surgical treatment groups

examined in these populations of patients to define markers for worse prognosis.

The presence of micrometastases detected by additional sectioning [24-26] did not show any significant prognostic value, although these observations were based on a small number of patients [26] or a short follow-up time [24,25]. Micrometastases detected by special stainings [27] have been shown to be an indicator of dire prognosis. This series, however, is also small. A trial of serial sectioning and identification of the prognostic value of small metastases, undetected by routine pathology examination, remains to be performed. Preliminary data from a recent trial show that the conversion rate from negative to positive (N- to N+) varies between 10% and 15%. It might be hypothesised that micrometastatic disease is the expression of an aggressive tumour which has been detected early, and that hence its observation carries an important prognostic value.

The interrelationship between the various prognostic factors described in Table 2 is still a matter of research. Most of these factors are related to one another. However, the chances are small that a patient would present with either *all* low-risk factors or *all* high-risk factors. The prognostic value added by each of the factors in one or in the other direction is as yet unknown.

Table 2. Prognostic variables in N- breast cancer populations

Prognostic factor	Low risk	High risk	Reference
Tumour size	≤ 2	≥ 2	7,10,11
Site of primary*		Internal quadrants	12,13
Nuclear grade	Good	Poor	8
Histological grade	Low (well differentiated)	High (poorly differentiated)	14
Labelling index	Low	High	15,16
Proliferation analysis	Diploid & low S-phase	Aneuploid or diploid with abundant S-phase	17
Oestrogen receptor content **	High	Low or none	5,18-20
Oncogene amplification and/or expression ***	Low	High	21-23

* Represents a controversy: small differences [12]
** Patients with ER- primaries have worse prognoses in all series. The magnitude of the difference is smaller for the majority of the series [18-20], which are also the ones more recently evaluated
*** Based upon very small numbers of patients; must still be confirmed

Trials of Adjuvant Therapy for Patients with N- Breast Cancer

Information concerning the treatment of patients with N- disease is available from two types of trials. One type included patients with either N+ of N- breast cancer in which identical therapies are applied and the analysis of treatment effects for the N- subpopulation is performed retrospectively. Although these trials provide some evidence of an advantage for the patients who received chemotherapy [28,7] or tamoxifen [29-31], we will focus upon the other type of trials in which therapy was prospectively assigned to patients with N- disease.

The trials which were retrospectively designed to answer treatment questions in patients with node-negative breast cancer are summarised in Table 3. The disease- or relapse-free survival percentages of the patients who received the systemic adjuvant therapy as compared to control are presented. Overall survival differences are either not reported or are not statistically significant for the majority of the trials.

In general, the results of these trials, especially those with a large number of patients, confirm that both chemotherapy and tamoxifen significantly prolong disease-free survival. To date, there is little evidence that this will translate into an overall survival advantage. In fact, early prolongation of disease-free survival has not always resulted in a prolonged overall survival (i.e., post-menopausal women with N+ breast cancer treated with chemotherapy alone). Follow-up for the majority of the trials for N- patients is, however, quite short so that the number of deaths observed is too small to provide meaningful results regarding mortality reduction.

Nevertheless, a longer period spent without disease recurrence is in itself a meritorious result, especially if the overall burden of toxic effects is low (e.g. as with tamoxifen or with a short course of chemotherapy). Comparisons of treatment effects for women with N+ breast cancer which consider the quality of life of the patients [39], have demonstrated that, following an initial period of three years, the early toxicity in the entire population is balanced against the longer disease-free survival, even if no overall survival benefit is observed.

Table 3. Trials of adjuvant systemic therapy in N- breast cancer

Trial [ref]	Therapy	No. patients; population	Year reported results	RFS or DFS Rx	Control	Significance
OSAKO [32]	LMF x 6	122 All	9	63%	60%	No*
Midlands [33]	LMF x 8 (low dose)	543	5	75%	74%	No**
Mainz [34]	CMF	175 All	5	82%	72%	No**
Vienna [35]	CFVbM x 8 (3 years)	128 All	5	86%	78%	No***
Cardiff [36]	VAC x 6	52 ER-	3	83%	71%	Yes**
Milan [37]	i.v. CMF x 12	90 ER-	5	87%	45%	Yes***
NSABP B-13 [38]	M --> F x 13	741 ER-	4	80%	71%	Yes**
ECOG [38]	INT 0011	422 ER- or ER+ if T > 3cm	3	84%	67%	Yes**
NSABP B-14 [38]	TAM x 5 yrs	2644 ER+	4	82%	77%	Yes**
Ludwig V [20]	i.v. CMF x 1 (periop. only)	1275 All	4	77%	71%	Yes****

*   Overall survival: significant difference, p=0.07
**   Overall survival: comparison not available
***   Overall survival: significant difference ≤ p=0.02
****   Overall survival: not significant

The most important observation from recent large-scale studies of patients with N- breast cancer is that the relapse rates for patients who receive no adjuvant therapy, even for those who have ER+ primaries, are higher than had been expected. It may therefore be asserted that issues of over-treatment are hardly germane since the chance of relapse for many selected node-negative patients is high.

The poorer than expected outcome and the steady increase in the proportion of patients whose disease is N- have contributed to the current uncertainty about the prognosis of patients who are being diagnosed as having N- breast cancer. It is essential, therefore, that these patients be managed within controlled clinical trials. For N- patients with ER+ disease, especially in postmenopausal age, a control might include tamoxifen treatment. Trials for patients whose primaries are classified as ER- might have adjuvant chemotherapy as treatment for the control group. For other subpopulations, surgical controls should perhaps be maintained. It must, however, be recognised that even for the group benefiting most from adjuvant therapy, the proportion of patients who enjoy improved survival is much lower than the proportion of patients who relapse and die despite treatment. To improve outcome and increase knowledge in this field, a more widespread acceptance (even approval) of participation in clinical trials is warranted [40].

N- Breast Cancer and the Media

On the 18th of May, 1988, four days before the opening of the 24th Annual Meeting of the American Society of Clinical Oncology, the U.S. NCI sent a clinical alert letter to physicians, informing them that big, NCI-sponsored trials (NSABP study B-13, NSABP study B-14 and Intergroup study INT 0011) carried out with selected populations of N- breast cancer patients were found to significantly prolong disease-free survival in the treated women as compared to the randomly allocated controls [38] (see also Table 3).

The letter concluded that adjuvant hormonal therapy or cytotoxic chemotherapy can have a meaningful impact on the natural history of N- breast cancer patients. Outside of a clinical setting the hormonal and chemotherapy treatment represent credible therapeutic options. The New York Times in its late edition of May 21, 1988, came with a first page headline saying: "Cancer Drug Therapy Urged For All After Breast Surgery." Describing this event (i.e., the presentation of data from NCI-sponsored programmes before any peer-reviewed journal ever published the data), the New York Times also wrote: "In issuing news on cancer, Institute chose mail, not media." Reading these articles one notes the following sentences: "Earlier this week the Institute announced the data in a letter to 13,000 doctors without waiting to publish the results in medical journals or to present them at a scientific meeting. It said the potential effect of its new findings was so great, that we wish to inform practicing physicians in advance of publication."

We describe the above events and the reaction to them by the media to illustrate that clinical trials and their results have an impact upon the social, political and economic spheres of medicine. The media response appeared to be one of emotional disappointment at having been "robbed" of the opportunity to publicise a significant medical progress. In fact, if some of this emotional energy would be devoted to make available clinical trials more widely known to the public and to advertise their social acceptability as the most appropriate means to provide the best available care, a much more significant medical progress would be made.

REFERENCES

1 Harris JR, Henderson IC: Natural history and staging of breast cancer. In: Harris JR, Hellman S, Henderson IC, Kinne DW (eds) Breast Diseases. JB Lippincott Co, Philadelphia 1987 pp 233-258

2 UK Trial of Early Detection of Breast Cancer Group. First results on mortality reduction in the UK trial of early detection of breast cancer. Lancet 1988 (ii):411-416

3 Ludwig Breast Cancer Study Group: Randomized perioperative therapy in operable breast cancer: the Ludwig Study V. Proc of the 3rd Conference on Adjuvant Therapy of Primary Breast Cancer. St Gallen 1988 p 8

4 Valagussa P, Bonadonna G, Veronesi U: Patterns of relapse and survival in operable breast carcinoma with positive and negative axillary nodes. Tumori 1978 (64):241-258

5 Valagussa P, Bignami P, Buzzoni R et al: Are estrogen receptors alone a reliable prognostic factor in node-negative breast cancer? In: Jones SE and Salmon SE (eds) Adjuvant Therapy of Cancer IV. Grune & Stratton, Orlando 1984 pp 407-415

6 Veronesi U, Saccozzi R, DelVecchio M et al: Comparing radical mastectomy with quadrantectomy, axillary dissection and radiotherapy in patients with small cancer of the breast. N Engl J Med 1981 (305):6-11

7 Fisher B, Slack N, Katrych D et al: Ten-year follow-up results of patients with carcinoma of the breast in a cooperative trial evaluating surgical adjuvant chemotherapy. Surg Gynecol Obstet 1975 (140):528-534

8 Fisher ER, Sass R, Fisher B: Pathological findings from the National Surgical Adjuvant Project for Breast Cancer (protocol #4). Cancer 1984 (53):712-723

9 Fisher B, Bauer M, Margolese R et al: Five-year results of a randomized clinical trial comparing total mastectomy and segmental mastectomy with or without radiation in the treatment of breast cancer. N Engl J Med 1985 (312):665-670

10 Valagussa P, Bonadonna G, Veronesi U: Patterns of relapse and survival following radical mastectomy. Cancer 1978 (41):1170-1178

11 Nemoto T, Vana J, Bedwani RN et al: Management and survival of female breast cancer: results of a national survey by the American College of Surgeons. Cancer 1980 (45):2917-2924

12 Handley RS: Carcinoma of the breast. Ann R Coll Surg Engl 1975 (57):59-66

13 Veronesi U, Cascinelli N, Greco M et al: Prognosis of breast cancer patients after mastectomy and dissection of internal mammary nodes. Ann Surg 1985 (202):702-707

14 Bloom HJG and Field JR: Impact of tumor grade and host resistance on survival of women with breast cancer. Cancer 1971 (28):1580-1589

15 Tubiana M, Pejovic MN, Chavandra N et al: The long term prognostic significance of the thymidine labeling index in breast cancer. Int J Cancer 1984 (30):441-445

16 Silvestrini R, Daidone MG and Gasparini G: Cell kinetics as a prognostic marker in node-negative breast cancer. Cancer 1985 (56):1982-1987

17 Dressler LG, Seamer LC, Owen MA et al: DNA flow cytometry and prognostic factors in 1331 frozen breast cancer specimens. Cancer 1988 (61):420-427

18 William MR, Todd JH, Ellis IO et al: Oestrogen receptors in primary and advanced breast cancer: an eight year review of 706 cases. Br J Cancer 1986 (55):67

19 Fisher B, Redmond C, Fisher ER et al: Relative worth of estrogen or progesterone receptor and pathologic characteristics of differentiation as indicators of prognosis in node-negative breast cancer patients: Findings from the NSABP protocol B-06. J Clin Oncol 1988 (6):1076-1087

20 Ludwig Breast Cancer Group: Ludwig Trial V Results (unpublished)

21 McGuire WL: The risk of recurrence in breast cancer patients. In: Proc of the 3rd International Conference on Adjuvant Therapy of Primary Breast Cancer. St Gallen 1988 p 19

22 Gullick WJ, Berger MS, Bennett PLP et al: Expression of the c-erbB-2 protein in normal and transformed cells. Int J Cancer 1987 (40):246-254

23 Hynes NE, Berger M, Locher G et al: Analysis of the c-erbB-2 proto-oncogene in human breast carcinomas: correlation of gene amplification, protein expression and clinical parameters. In: Proc of the 3rd International Conference on Adjuvant Therapy of Primary Breast Cancer. St Gallen 1988 p 4

24 Hovus AG, Hutter RVP, Berg JW: Significance of axillary macrometastases and micrometastases in mammary cancer. Ann Surg 1971 (173):44-46

25 Fisher ER, Swamidoss S, Lee CH et al: Detection and significance of occult axillary node metastases in patients with invasive breast cancer. Cancer 1978 (42):2025-2031

26 Rosen PP, Saigo PE, Brown DW Jr et al: Prognosis in stage II (T1N1M0) breast cancer. Ann Surg 1981 (194):576-581

27 Benchabbat A, Friedman S, Mouziesse H et al: Clandestine metastasis of breast axillary lymph nodes: A finding confirming worse prognosis than standard nodal metastasis. In: Proc ECCO 4, Madrid 1987 p113

28 Nissen-Meyer R, Kjellgren K, Malmio K et al: Surgical adjuvant chemotherapy. Results with one short course of cyclophosphamide after mastectomy for breast cancer. Cancer 1978 (41):2088-2098

29 Nolvadex Adjuvant Trial Organisation: Controlled trial of tamoxifen as a single adjuvant agent in the management of early breast cancer. Br J Cancer 1988 (57):608-611

30 Scottish Cancer Trials Office: Adjuvant tamoxifen in the management of operable breast cancer. The Scottish trial. Lancet 1987 (ii):171-175

31 CRC Adjuvant Breast Trial Working Party. Cyclophosphamide and tamoxifen as adjuvant therapies in the management of breast cancer. Br J Cancer 1988 (57):604-607

32 Senn HJ, Jungi WF, Amgwerd R et al: Swiss adjuvant trial (OSAKO 06/74) with chlorambucil, methotrexate

and 5-fluorouracil plus BCG in node-negative breast cancer patients: five-year results. NCI Monographs 1986 (1):129-134

33 Morrison JM, Howell A, Grieve RJ et al: The West Midlands Oncology Association trials on adjuvant chemotherapy for operable breast cancer. In: Salmon SE (ed): Adjuvant Therapy of Cancer V. Grune & Stratton, Orlando 1987 pp 311-318

34 Caffier H, Rotte K, Haeggqwist O: Adjuvant chemotherapy versus postoperative irradiation in node-negative breast cancer. In: Jones SE and Salmon SE (eds) Adjuvant Therapy of Cancer IV. Grune & Stratton, Orlando 1984 pp 417-424

35 Jakesz R, Kolb R, Reiner G et al: Adjuvant chemotherapy in node-negative breast cancer patients. In: Salmon SE (ed): Adjuvant Therapy of Cancer V. Grune & Stratton, Orlando 1987 pp 223-231

36 Williams CJ, Buchanan RB, Hall V et al: Adjuvant chemotherapy for T_{1-2}, N_1, M_0 estrogen receptor negative breast cancer: preliminary results of a randomized trial. In: Salmon SE (ed): Adjuvant Therapy of Cancer V. Grune & Stratton, Orlando 1987 pp 233-241

37 Bonadonna G, Valagussa P, Zambetti M et al: Milan adjuvant trials for stage I-II breast cancer. In: Salmon SE (ed): Adjuvant Therapy of Cancer V. Grune & Stratton, Orlando 1987 pp 211-221

38 NEWS FROM NCI: Treatment alert issues for node-negative breast cancer. JNCI 1988 (80):550-551

39 Goldhirsch A, Gelber RD, Simes RJ et al: Costs and benefits of adjuvant therapy in breast cancer: a quality adjusted survival analysis. J Clin Oncol 1989 (in press)

40 Gelber RD, Goldhirsch A: Can a clinical trial be the treatment of choice for patients with cancer? JNCI 1988 (80):886-887

New Developments in the Field of Aromatase Inhibitors

F. Cavalli

Division of Oncology, Ospedale San Giovanni, 6500 Bellinzona, Switzerland

Introduction

Oestrogens play the most important role in maintaining the growth of established breast cancer. Therefore, suppression of circulating plasma levels of oestrogens may induce regression of tumour growth. In premenopausal women the ovaries are the main source of oestrogens, while in postmenopausal women oestrogens are mainly derived from extra-ovarian aromatisation of androgenic precursors such as androstenedione [1].

The role of aromatase, a microsomal cytochrome P-450 dependent enzyme system, is well established as a key enzyme in the biosynthesis of oestrogens in males and females [2]. Aromatase is found predominantly in the premenopausal ovary and also in adipose tissue, liver, brain, placenta and breast cancer tissue [3,4].

The development of inhibitors of aromatase has been a matter of considerable interest since the pioneering studies of Schwarzel et al. [5] in 1973. Among many other aromatase inhibitors, aminoglutethimide is the only one which has successfully entered medical practice in the treatment of advanced breast cancer.

Aminoglutethimide: A Review

Aminoglutethimide (AG), derived from a non-barbiturate soporific and originally introduced as an anticonvulsant drug, was subsequently discovered to inhibit steroidogenesis (Fig. 1). As early as 1966 Schteingard et al. reported successful control in a patient with functional disseminated adrenocortical carcinoma [6]. At that time it was still unknown that it interferes with the aromatisation of androstenedione. Nevertheless, it was already introduced in the palliative treatment of advanced breast cancer in 1967 [7] but it was only many years later, when its mechanism of action was clarified [8,9], that this drug could be used in an optimal manner [10,11]. Usually AG is administered with hydrocortisone to prevent a reflex rise in pituitary ACTH. The endocrine effects of aminoglutethimide plus hydrocortisone were reviewed recently [12]. This is an important topic, since substantial clinical improvement in advanced breast cancer has been reported on corticoids alone [13,14]. The paper of Alexieva-Figusch [12] shows that the endocrine effects of administration of the combination AG and hydrocortisone differ from those of hydrocortisone alone. Because of the large suppression of "free" oestradiol levels, the combination may be superior to the effect of the single drugs in the treatment of metastatic breast cancer. This has been confirmed recently in a clinical trial comparing low-dose AG with or without hydrocortisone: the combination showed a statistically significant superiority in response rate and time to progression [15]. AG produces approximately 30% tumour regression in postmenopausal patients [10,11], while in premenopausal women its activity still has to be clearly defined. The response rate to aminoglutethimide is therefore very similar to the therapeutic results which can be achieved in the treatment of advanced breast cancer with all types of effective endocrine treatment [16]. In comparison mainly with Tamoxifen, AG shows a more pronounced toxicity and is therefore

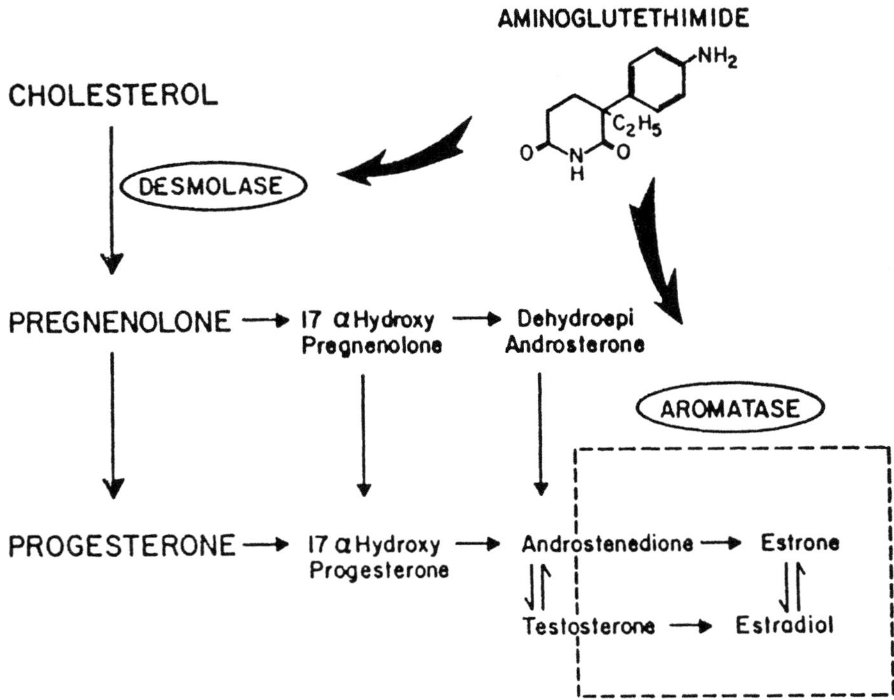

Fig. 1. Mechanism of action of Aminoglutethimide

more difficult to handle. Acute toxicity, mainly related to the soporific effect of AG, may be present in up to 50% of the patients. However, with continued treatment this toxicity disappears in most patients [10,11,16-19]. In about 7-10% of the patients the treatment has to be interrupted mainly due to chronic toxicity (depression, muscle cramps etc.). Several studies have attempted to evaluate the hypothesis that a lower dose of AG would produce less side effects. In a French study 150 patients were randomised to receive either 500 mg or 1 g of AG plus hydrocortisone: the response rates were similar in both arms and there was an indication of better tolerance with the lower dosage [20]. However, in a dose-escalation study, low doses of AG were shown to be active, but the frequency of side effects was similar to that with conventional doses [21].

In 2 studies [17,18], the response to prior Tamoxifen was shown to correlate with an increased probability of activity of AG. Conversely, low response rates were observed with Tamoxifen in patients previously treated with AG [17,19]. AG may therefore be a better second-line treatment in advanced breast cancer than Tamoxifen. Moreover, in a phase II trial with AG in advanced postmenopausal breast carcinoma carried out by the Swiss Group for Clinical Cancer Research (SAKK), a comparison of patients with and without prior medroxyprogesterone acetate showed a significant difference in the response rate to the immediately following treatment with AG plus hydrocortisone: 4% versus 32%, p = 0.02 [22]. These observations raise the question of a possible interaction among different endocrine agents and of the optimal sequence in the hormonal management of patients with advanced breast cancer. These problems have been extensively reviewed in the first volume of this Monograph [23]. As with most effective endocrine agents, higher response rates may be achieved with AG in the presence of predictive factors such as skin or soft-tissue metastases, a long disease-free interval from surgery to tumour reappearance and positive tumour receptors. Table 1 summarises the results in different series of

Table 1. Results in different series of patients treated with second-line aminoglutethimide

Reference	[7]	[6]	[11]	[27]	[22]	[26]	[25]	[24]
No. of patients	91	129	190	52	42	67	38	85
CR + PR (%)								
a) Total series	33	37	28	19	14	13.4	13	17
b) Site of lesions								
Viscera	34	29	18.8	15	10	21	22	14.7
Bone	29.6	35	23	0	0	14.6	13	3.8
Soft tissue	0	47	30	29	13	10	6	40.7
Duration of response, median in months	11	14	14	4.5	10.5	7	12.5	11

patients treated with second-line AG also with regard to the site of the lesions.

Currently the results correlating antitumour activity of AG and tumour level of aromatase are scanty and inconsistent.

Other Aromatase Inhibitors

Since AG is not selective in its inhibition of aromatase and has shown consistent clinical toxicity, there has been an intensive search for other aromatase inhibitors. So far, only a few have undergone clinical evaluation. Trilostane (4a 5 epoxy-17 ß-hydroxy-3-oxo 5 a androstane-2-carbonitrile) is an effective inhibitor of the 3ß-hydroxysteroid dehydrogenase, $\Delta 5$-4 isomerase system in the rat adrenal, inhibiting the conversion of the biologically inactive $\Delta 5$ steroids to their $\Delta 4$ derivatives [28]. In a study involving 23 postmenopausal patients with advanced breast cancer, Trilostane showed a response rate of 26% [29]. A similar result was found in a study carried out by the SAKK [30]. Overall, trilostane not only has a mechanism of action which apparently resembles that of AG, but it also produces therapeutic results and side effects that are very similar to those observed with AG. Another derivative which has undergone some clinical evaluation is 4-hydroxyandrostenedione (4-OHA). It has been shown that 4-OHA is not only a more potent inhibitor

of aromatase as compared to aminoglutethimide, it is also much more selective, since it does not inhibit cortisol synthesis and thus steroid replacement is not needed. During the clinical evaluation of 4-OHA it was shown that it had a remarkable lack of side effects [31]. The major disadvantage of 4-OHA is the need for parenteral administration, mainly since it involves some pain at the injection site. Recently the results of a phase II study involving 65 postmenopausal patients with advanced breast cancer were published: the response rate was 27%, while the side effects were mostly nonspecific and of low intensity [32]. Notwithstanding the fact that this drug has shown clinical activity, its use has therefore been limited in the last years because of this formulation problem.

New Aromatase Inhibitors

In recent years there has been an extensive search for more selective aromatase inhibitors of higher potency, and various compounds are either at the end of their preclinical evaluation or entering clinical studies. In the last few years we have been working with CGS 16949A (see Fig. 2), which is a new non-steroidal inhibitor of aromatase with higher potency and much greater specificity in its inhibition of aromatase than AG [33]. This was shown both *in vitro* [34] and *in vivo* [33].

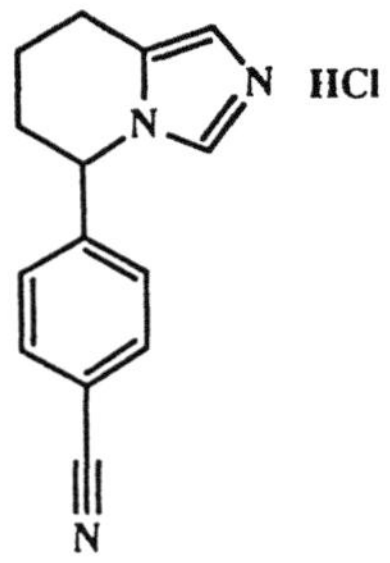

Fig. 2. Structure of CGS 16 949 A

In vitro CGS 16949A is 100 times more potent than AG in inhibiting aromatase, *in vivo* it is about 1,000 times more potent than AG in blocking the conversion of androgens to oestrogens. Given orally to rats it interrupts cyclicity, suppresses oestradiol and shows marked anti-tumour activity in DMBA-induced mammary tumours. At the maximum aromatase inhibiting concentration it does not reduce adrenal steroidogenesis in animals. We treated 23 postmenopausal patients with advanced measurable breast cancer. The drug was given p.o. t.i.d. for at least 30 days: 0.1 mg in 7 patients, 0.2 mg in 6 patients and 0.3 mg in 10 patients. The treatment was perfectly well tolerated and we saw only nonspecific and minor dose-independent side effects.

In this study anti-tumour activity was seen in at least 2 patients with measurable disease [35]. Similar results were reported recently by 2 other groups [36,37]. Because of these encouraging preliminary results, various phase II trials have been activated recently. In particular in one study, undertaken by the Swiss Group for Clinical Cancer Research (SAKK), CGS 16949A is compared to Tamoxifen in postmenopausal patients with advanced breast cancer previously unexposed to endocrine agents.

Conclusions

Aromatase inhibition is not only a fascinating biological topic, but also a very promising lead for more active treatments against breast cancer. Up till now the importance of this type of endocrine treatment has been somewhat limited by the toxicity of first-generation compounds such as AG. At present new compounds with a higher potency and a greater selectivity are under clinical evaluation. The preliminary results are very promising; it is, therefore, likely that in the next years this field will become much more important than it has been in the past. Clinical results are therefore eagerly awaited.

REFERENCES

1 Poortman J, Thijssen JHH, Schwarz F: Androgen production and conversion to estrogens in normal postmenopausal women and in selected breast cancer patients. J Clin Endocrinol Metab 1973 (37):101-109

2 Fishman J: Biochemical mechanism of aromatization. Cancer Res 1982 (42 Suppl):3277s-3280s

3 Schindler AE, Ebert A, Friedrich EF: Conversion of androstenedione to estrone by human fat tissue. J Clin Endocrinol Metab 1972 (35):627-630

4 Nimrod A and Ryan K: Aromatization of androgens by human abdominal and breast fat tissue. J Clin Endocrinol Metab 1975 (40):362-372

5 Schwarzel WC, Kruggel W, Brodie HJ: The development of inhibitors of the enzyme system in human placenta. Endocrinol 1973 (92):866-880

6 Schteingard GE, Cash R, Conn JW: Aminoglutethimide and metastatic adrenal cancer. J Am Med Assoc 1966 (198):1007-1010

7 Gale KE: Treatment of advanced breast cancer with aminoglutethimide: a 14-year experience. Cancer Res 1982 (42 Suppl):3389s-3396s

8 Salhanick HA: Basic studies on aminoglutethimide. Cancer Res 1982 (42 Suppl):3315s-3321s

9 Abdul-Hajj YJ: Comparative studies of aromatase inhibitors in relation to the significance of estrogen synthesis in human mammary tumors. Cancer Res 1982 (42 Suppl):3373s-3377s

10 Santen RJ, Wotgul TJ, Lipton A et al: Aminoglutethimide as treatment of postmenopausal women with advanced breast carcinoma. Ann Intern Med 1982 (96):94-101

11 Harris AI, Powles TJ, Smith IF: Aminoglutethimide in the treatment of advanced postmenopausal breast cancer. Cancer Res 1982 (42 Suppl):3405s-3408s

12 Alexieva-Figusch J, De Jong FH, Lamberts SWJ, Van Gilse HA, Klijn JGM: Endocrine effects of aminoglutethimide plus hydrocortisone versus effects of high dose of hydrocortisone alone in postmenopausal metastatic breast cancer. Eur J Cancer Clin Oncol 1987 (23):1349-1356

13 Jakobsen A, Frederiksen PL, Möller KAA et al: Medroxyprogesterone acetate and prednisone in advanced breast cancer. A randomized trial. Eur J Cancer Clin Oncol 1986 (22):1067-1073

14 Van Gilse HA: Long-term treatment with corticosteroids of patients with metastatic breast cancer. Cancer Chemother Rep 1962 (16):293-298

15 Bisani G, Cocconi G, Ceci G, Franciosi V, Bartolucci R, Gori S, Carpi A, Passalacqua R, Bacchi M: Aminoglutethimide (AG) a bassa dose, con o senza idrocortisone (HC) come prima linea endocrina nel carcinoma avanzato della mammella. Studio prospettico e randomizzato del Goirc. Tumori 1987 (73 Suppl):86

16 Mouridsen HT: Endocrine treatment of advanced breast cancer. In: Cavalli F (ed) Endocrine Therapy of Breast Cancer: Concepts and Strategies. ESO Monograph Series, Springer Verlag, Berlin 1986 pp 79-90

17 Smith IF, Harris AI, Morgan M, Gazet JC, McKinna JA: Tamoxifen versus aminoglutethimide versus combined tamoxifen and aminoglutethimide in the treatment of advanced breast carcinoma. Cancer Res 1982 (42 Suppl):3430s-3432s

18 Murray RMI, Pitt P: Aminoglutethimide in tamoxifen-resistant patients: The Melbourne experience. Cancer Res 1982 (42 Suppl):3437s-3438s

19 Santen RJ: Experience with aminoglutethimide in 147 postmenopausal mammary carcinoma patients. Clinical results and plasma steroid values. In: Paesi FJR (ed) Aminoglutethimide (Orimeten). Mechanism of Action and Clinical Results in Breast Cancer. Ciba-Geigy, Basle 1982 pp 11-34

20 Bonneterre J, Coppens H, Mauriac L, Metz M, Rouesse J, Armand JP, Fargeot P, Mathieu M, Tubiana M, Cappelaere P: Aminoglutethimide in advanced breast cancer: Clinical results of a French multicenter randomized trial comparing 500 mg and 1 g/day. Eur J Clin Oncol 1985 (21):1153-1158

21 Stuart-Harris R, Bozek T, Gazet JC, Kurkure A, Dowsett M, McKinna JA, Jeffcoate SL, Carr L, Smith IE: Low dose aminoglutethimide in treatment of advanced breast cancer. Lancet 1984 (2):604-607

22 Alberto P, Mermillod B, Kaplan E, Goldhirsch A, Obrecht JP, Jungi F, Martz G, Barrelet L, Cavalli F: A clinical trial of aminoglutethimide in advanced postmenopausal breast carcinoma: Low response in patients previously treated with medroxyprogesterone. Eur J Cancer Clin Oncol 1985 (21):423-428

23 Gelber RD and Goldhirsch A: Methodology of clinical trials. investigating endocrine mechanisms in breast cancer. In: Cavalli F (ed) Endocrine Therapy of Breast Cancer: Concepts and Strategies. ESO Monograph Series, Springer Verlag, Berlin 1986 pp 51-78

24 Zambetti S, Brambilla C, Tancini G, Bonadonna G: Aminoglutethimide in postmenopausal breast cancer refractory to multiple hormonal and cytostatic treatments. Tumori 1987 (73):369-373

25 Höffken K, Kempf H, Miller AA, Miller B, Schmidt CG, Faber P, Kley HK: Aminoglutethimide without hydrocortisone in the treatment of post-menopausal patients with advanced breast cancer. Cancer Treat Rep 1986 (70):1153-1157

26 Pronzato P, Ardizzoni A, Lionetto R, Conte P, Rosso R: Aminoglutethimide as second-line endocrine treatment in metastatic breast cancer. Tumori 1985 (71):297-300

27 Kaye SB, Woods RL, Fox RM, Coates AS, Tattersall HN: Use of aminoglutethimide as second-line endocrine therapy in metastatic breast cancer. Cancer Res 1982 (42 Suppl): 3445-3447

28 Potts GO, Creange JE, Harding HR, Schane HP: Trilostane, an orally active inhibitor of steroid biosynthesis. Steroids 1978 (32):257

29 Beardwell CG, Hindley AC, Wilkinson PM, Todd IDH, Ribeiro GG, Bu'Lock D: Trilostane in the treatment of advanced breast cancer. Cancer Chemother and Pharmacol 1983 (10):158-160

30 Senn HJ, Varini M: unpublished results

31 Coombes RC, Dowsett M, Goss PE, Gazett JC, Brodie A: 4-hydroxyandrostenedione in treatment of

postmenopausal patients with advanced breast cancer. Lancet 1984 (2):1237-1239

32 Hoeffken A, Jonath W, Bossinger K, Kölbel M, Kunz T, Becher R, Callies R: Aromatase inhibition with 4-hydroxyandrostenedione (4-OHA) in the treatment of postmenopausal advanced breast cancer. Proceedings 13th Congress of ESMO, 1988, abstract No 180

33 Schieweck K, Bhatnagar AS, Matter A: CGS 16949A, a new non-steroidal aromatase inhibitor: Effects on hormone-dependent and independent tumors in vivo. Cancer Res 1988 (48):834-838

34 Steele RE, Mellor L, Sawyer WK, Wasvary JM, Browne LJ: In vitro and in vivo studies demonstrating potent and selective estrogen inhibition with the nonsteroidal aromatase inhibitor CGS 16949A. Steroids 1988 (in press)

35 Beretta K, Willems Y, Nadjafi C, Sessa C, Cavalli F: Phase I-II study in postmenopausal patients with advanced breast cancer of CGS 16949A: a new highly potent and selective aromatase inhibitor. Proceedings 13th Congress of ESMO, 1988, abstract No 181

36 Lipton A, Harvey HA, Demers LM, Hanagan J, Mulagha M, Sanders S, Fritzsimmons S, Santen RJ: A phase I trial of CGS 16949A - A new aromatase inhibitor. Proceedings 13th Congress of ESMO, 1988, abstract No 125

37 Stein RC, Davenport J, Hedley A, Coombes RC: Preliminary study of CGS 16949A in advanced postmenopausal breast cancer. Proceedings 13th Congress of ESMO, 1988, abstract No 182

Resistance to Antioestrogen Therapy: a Challenge for the Future

V. Craig Jordan

Department of Human Oncology, University of Wisconsin Clinical Cancer Center, Madison, Wisconsin 53792, U.S.A.

The Current Clinical Situation

Tamoxifen (Nolvadex®) is the first-line endocrine therapy for advanced breast cancer. About 30% of unselected patients have an objective response, although another 20% have stable disease. If oestrogen receptor-positive patients are selected for study, tamoxifen produces a 50-60% objective response rate. Nevertheless, about 13% of oestrogen receptor-negative patients can have a response to therapy.

Aside from the effectiveness of antioestrogen therapy, one of the keys to the success of tamoxifen is the low incidence of reported side effects [1]. This fact was important for the application as an adjuvant therapy in stage I/II breast cancer. Short term (2 years) of adjuvant tamoxifen therapy of stage II breast cancer has shown some benefits either with [3], or without [4] combination chemotherapy. However, based upon laboratory evidence which demonstrates that tamoxifen should be given indefinitely [5], trials of long-term adjuvant therapy show the advantage of prolonged therapy [6,7,8 plus ECOG unpublished data]. Indeed, tamoxifen has recently been shown to be effective in both pre- and post-menopausal women with stage I disease (NSABP protocol B14 unpublished results). As a result, the National Cancer Institute of the United States has recently (May 1988) issued a clinical alert to advise all medical oncologists to consider treatment of oestrogen receptor-positive stage I breast cancer patients with tamoxifen.

The value of long-term adjuvant tamoxifen therapy is becoming clear with successive publications from major clinical trial organisations. Tamoxifen therapy has proved to be safe and effective, however, not all patients with oestrogen receptor-positive breast tumours respond and therapy that is initially successful, eventually fails. To build on the initial success of tamoxifen therapy, it is important to understand the mechanisms of therapeutic failure in order to develop additional therapeutic strategies to apply when resistance to tamoxifen occurs.

The aim of this chapter is to propose various mechanisms for resistance to tamoxifen therapy and review some of the laboratory models that are currently being used to understand the environments that will subvert antioestrogen action. The potential mechanisms that will be considered are:
1. Metabolic tolerance
2. Hormone-independent (oestrogen receptor-negative) growth
3. Endocrine-regulated cell growth
4. Tamoxifen-dependent growth.

Metabolic Tolerance

Tamoxifen is extensively metabolised in animals and man [1,2]. The principal metabolic alterations are to form either 4-hydroxytamoxifen, which has a higher affinity for the oestrogen receptor and in some test systems is a more potent antioestrogen [9], or alterations in the side chain of tamoxifen to form N-desmethyltamoxifen, the principal metabolite in patients [10], and Metabolite Y [11] (Fig. 1). Each of the metabolites described have antioestrogenic properties in test systems so that the actions of tamoxifen as an antitumour agent can be considered to

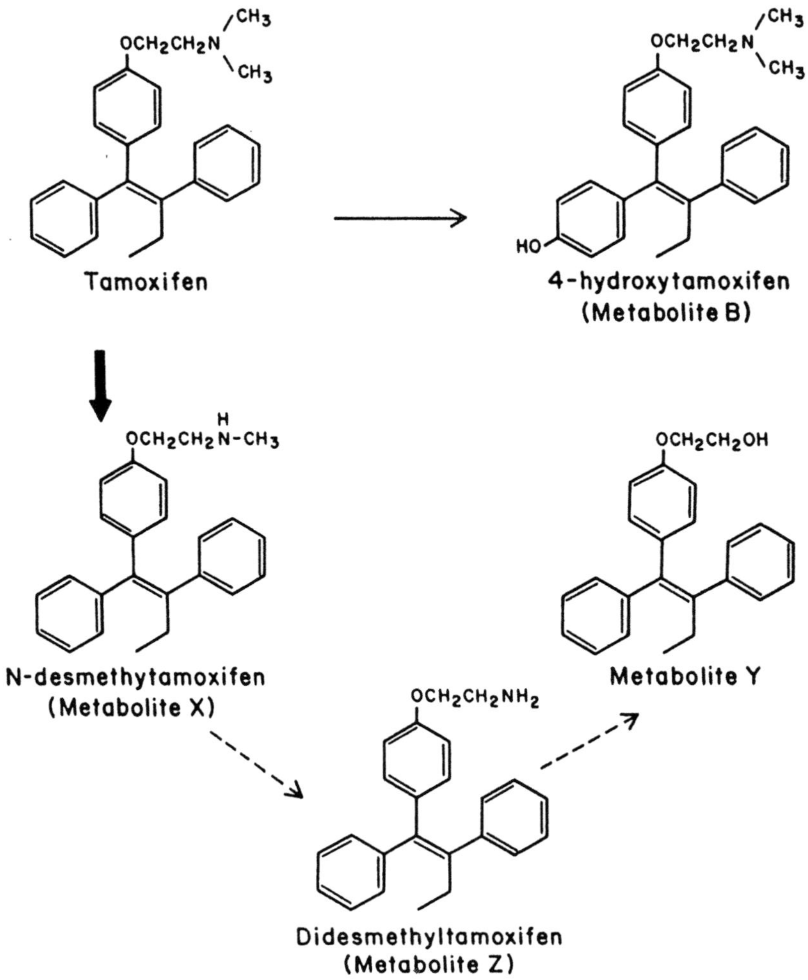

Tamoxifen

4-hydroxytamoxifen
(Metabolite B)

N-desmethytamoxifen
(Metabolite X)

Metabolite Y

Didesmethyltamoxifen
(Metabolite Z)

Fig. 1. The metabolism of tamoxifen in animals and man

be a combination of the effects of the parent drugs and its metabolites.

However, tamoxifen has some intriguing species-specific effects. Tamoxifen is an oestrogen in short-term assays using mice [1] and the drug has oestrogenic properties in the dog [1]. In fact, an oestrogenic metabolite of tamoxifen, Metabolite E (tamoxifen without the dimethylaminoethyl side chain), has been identified in dog bile, which naturally led to the possibility that the species differences might be because differential metabolic pathways are present. To date no evidence for this hypothesis has been found [12,13]. Indeed, the idea that tamoxifen is an oestrogen in the mouse may need to be modified with the recent findings that long-term tamoxifen therapy produces complete antioestrogenic effects in the mouse uterus. There is an initial stimulation of uterine tissues (1-2 months) then followed by a completely refractory phase [14]. This may be similar to the initial tumour stimulation (tumour flare) noted in patients before tamoxifen produces an effect. These data also point to the need to determine the effects of long-term tamoxifen therapy upon the human uterus. A quiescent uterine endometrium would obviously be an advantage.

There is only one study [6] of the levels of circulating metabolites of tamoxifen during adjuvant therapy for up to 5 years. No changes in the metabolic profile have been noted although one case of non-compliance was detected [15] which possibly resulted in recurrence of the disease. Currently we are surveying our patients who have successfully completed up to 10 years of tamoxifen therapy.

In summary, the idea that metabolic tolerance to tamoxifen might develop during long-term

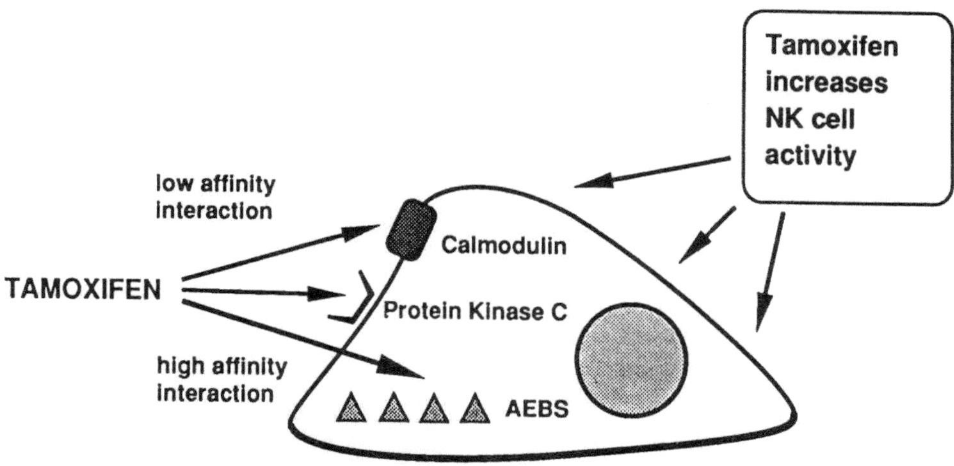

Fig. 2. Possible nonoestrogen receptors mediate actions of tamoxifen on breast cancer cells

therapy which then causes therapeutic failure, is not supported by studies completed to date.

Hormone Independent (Oestrogen Receptor Negative) Growth

It is almost axiomatic to believe that oestrogen receptor negative tumours are unable to respond to antioestrogen action in the absence of the oestrogen receptor system. However, up to 13% of tumours that are designated oestrogen receptor negative exhibit an objective response to tamoxifen. Although these tumours may be classified incorrectly by the receptor laboratory (poor sample procurement and techniques), alternate mechanisms for antioestrogen action may be present. These are illustrated in Figure 2. Most of these biochemical mechanisms (that depend upon high local concentrations of tamoxifen to produce an effect) have been reviewed [16]. Of interest is the possibility that natural killer (NK) cell activity in patients might be altered to facilitate tumour cell destruction. One report [17] indicates that this is a possibility but the correct experiments have not been done. A long-term evaluation of the effects of tamoxifen during adjuvant therapy is necessary. Indeed it is possible that there is an early positive effect of tamoxifen on NK cell activity but this declines with extended therapy. This phenomenon could possibly contribute to the failure of tamoxifen in some receptor-negative patients.

Endocrine Regulated Cell Growth

a) Oestrogens

Oestrogens stimulate the growth of breast cancer cells through the oestrogen receptor system. Clinical trials have demonstrated the value of using the measurement of oestrogen receptors to predict the success of endocrine therapy for breast cancer [for a review see 18]. At the subcellular level, the model for oestrogen action has evolved in recent years to incorporate current theories of cell replication through the release or activation of autocrine growth factors (Fig. 3). Indeed it is possible that oestrogens not only increase the availability of stimulatory growth factors (transforming growth factor alpha and insulin-like growth factor) but also decrease the availability of inhibitory growth factors like transforming growth factor beta [19].

Antioestrogens such as tamoxifen block oestrogen binding to the nuclear oestrogen receptor to decrease the availability of TGF alpha and IGF and to increase the availability of TGF beta (Fig. 4). The overall effect is to cause a blockade in the G1 phase of the breast cancer cell cycle [20].

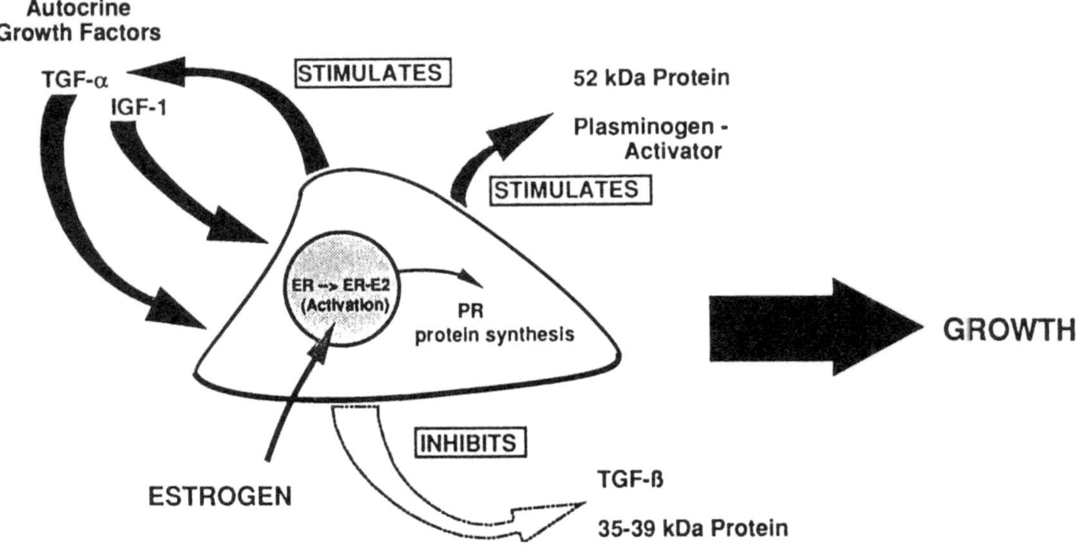

Fig. 3. Oestrogen-mediated effects in breast cancer cells

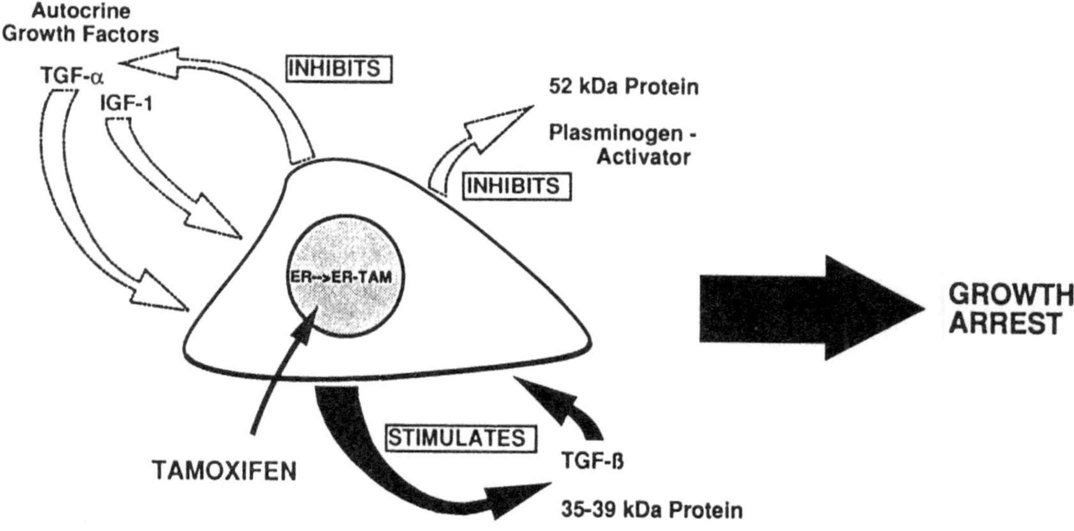

Fig. 4. The inhibition of oestrogen-stimulated growth in breast cancer cells by tamoxifen

Since tamoxifen and its metabolites are competitive inhibitors of oestrogen action then clinical situations where high concentrations of circulating oestrogen are present may not be in the best interest of long-term therapeutic control. Patient compliance during long-term adjuvant therapy may become an issue if 5 or 10 years of tamoxifen becomes the standard for stage I/II disease. Once drug concentrations drop in the premenopausal patient then oestrogen may reactivate the quiescent disease. Alternatively it is known that tamoxifen can cause elevations in circulating oestrogen in premenopausal patients with advanced breast cancer. Tamoxifen is known to have efficacy and to be equivalent to oophorectomy [21,22]; however, patients who initially respond and then fail tamoxifen therapy may have a further response to oophorectomy [23]. It is possible that ovarian factors (oestrogen or progesterone) can re-activate growth in the tumour in spite of compliant tamoxifen therapy.

Similarly, long-term adjuvant tamoxifen therapy of young premenopausal women, following chemotherapy for stage II disease, results in elevated steroidogenesis in those women who continue to menstruate (Fig. 5A and B) [24]. Strategies to reduce steroidogenesis (Zoladex® administration) may prove to be of benefit to these patients and reduce the likelihood of tamoxifen failure.

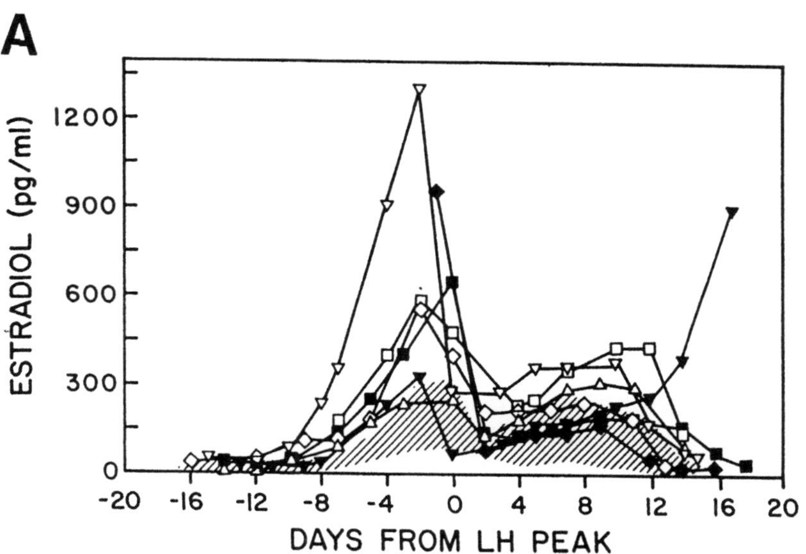

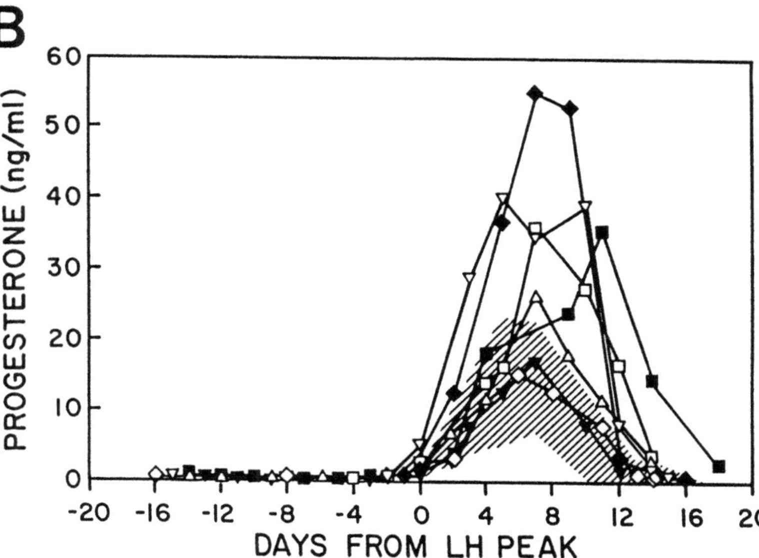

Fig. 5. The increase in A oestradiol and B progesterone observed in young premenopausal patients following adjuvant chemotherapy, but during long-term adjuvant tamoxifen therapy. The shaded areas represent the range for normal women

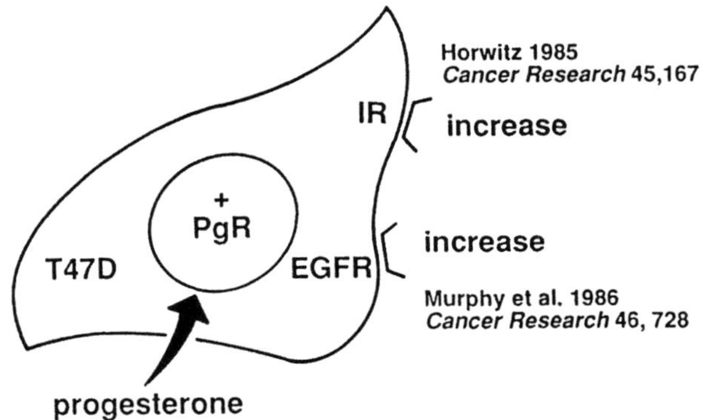

Fig. 6. Regulation of autocrine growth factor receptor by progesterone or progestational agents

b) Progesterone

The action of progesterone in oestrogen target tissues appears to be a paradox. It is well recognised that large doses of progestational agents exert an antioestrogenic action in the uterus, and this action has been employed to justify the use of high doses of progestational agents as a breast cancer therapy. However, the action of small doses of progestational agents is less well understood. At the subcellular level, progestational agents have been shown to alter the expression of growth factor receptors (Fig. 6) and progesterone can cause a slight increase in breast cancer cell replication *in vitro* [25]. It is possible that physiological concentrations of progesterone cause replication of breast tissues. Indeed the content of progestational agents in oral contraceptives has been linked with the genesis of breast cancer [26].

The question arises "Will the increased secretion of progesterone during tamoxifen therapy have a beneficial or harmful effect upon the control of breast cancer cell replication?" Two pieces of information suggest that progestational agents may have a negative effect upon the control of breast cancer cell replication by tamoxifen. The evaluation of a combination of low-dose progestational agent with tamoxifen was found to be *less* effective for the treatment of advanced breast cancer than tamoxifen alone [27]. Similarly, in the DMBA-induced rat mammary carcinoma model, the administration of daily injection of progesterone to tamoxifen-treated rats causes a reactivation of tumorigenesis [28]. An antiprogestin and an antioestrogen were superior to the antioestrogen alone in a progesterone-rich environment [28]. If these data can be extrapolated to the long-term adjuvant treatment of premenopausal patients with tamoxifen, increased secretion of ovarian progesterone may produce a less than optimal environment. Again, ovarian suppression would avoid any potential problems with excessive steroidogenesis.

c) Prolactin

Rat mammary tumours are known to show dependence upon prolactin for growth, however, the case for the prolactin dependence of human breast cancer is controversial and has been difficult to support therapeutically. Nevertheless, recent laboratory results [29] indicate that a variant of the MCF-7 breast cancer cell line can respond to human prolactin with a growth response but only in the absence of bovine prolactin in the serum-supplemented culture media. It appears that bovine prolactin can block human prolactin receptors but is unable to initiate a growth response. Thus, in the presence of bovine prolactin the action of human prolactin is inhibited.

Whilst the authors concede [29] that only one variant of MCF-7 cells was found to perform the appropriate response to prolactin, it does raise the question of whether prolactin could stimulate the growth of an ER-positive cell that was held in the G1 phase by an antioestrogen. Obviously if this was established then therapeutic measures that can increase prolactin (tranquillizers and antiemetics) may not be beneficial to the patient on long-term adjuvant tamoxifen therapy.

Overall, a variety of endocrine mechanisms may be able to reverse the effects of tamoxifen. These, in concert with the paracrine influences of growth factors in neighbouring cells, may be able to maintain the replication of receptor-positive cells during long-term tamoxifen therapy (Fig. 7).

Paracrine Regulated Cell Growth

Oestrogen may increase cell replication of oestrogen receptor positive cells by an increased activation or secretion of growth factors. In contrast, receptor-negative cells

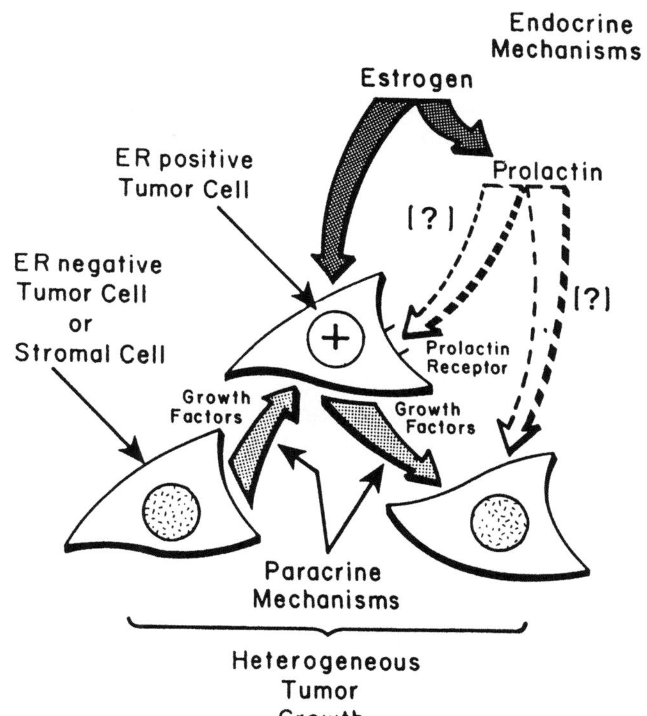

Fig. 7. Regulation of heterogeneous tumour growth through endocrine and paracrine mechanisms

may have an increased constituitive synthesis of growth factors. Indeed transfection of MCF-7 breast cancer cells with v-ras^H produces a cell line that is hormone independent for growth in athymic mice [30] and has a high constituitive production of growth factors [31]. However, the precise change from a cloned hormone-dependent breast cancer cell to a hormone-independent (oestrogen receptor negative) cell has not been documented in the laboratory. Several studies [32,33] have shown that oestrogen-deprived MCF-7 cells can increase their growth rate during long-term culture, but the oestrogen receptor is not lost. It is possible that a whole variety of chance events within the correct environment must come together to cause the adaptation of the cells *in vivo*. It is becoming clear that the paracrine influences of growth factors from adjacent cells, be they other breast cancer cells or stromal cells within the tumour matrix (Fig. 7), can alter the dynamics of cell replication of receptor positive cells.

This knowledge necessitates the consideration of a potential mechanism of tamoxifen resistance. If tamoxifen, or its metabolites, prevent cell replication by suppressing the production or activation of stimulatory growth factors, then a supply of growth factors from adjacent cells (paracrine) might activate cell replication of the tamoxifen blocked cell. Evidence is available using MCF-7 and T47D breast cancer cells [34-36] that the addition of epidermal growth factor can partially reverse the action of tamoxifen. Indeed the co-culture of MCF-7 cells and MDA-MB-231 cells (oestrogen receptor negative) using Costar transwells has demonstrated that factor from the MDA-MB-231 cells will cause the cell division of MCF-7 cells even in the presence of a variety of antioestrogens at concentrations which inhibit oestradiol stimulated growth [37].

Clearly these experiments have important clinical implications for an understanding of why antioestrogens only control the growth of a minority of tumours. Tumours are heterogeneous mixtures of receptor-positive and -negative cancer cells with different amounts of stromal tissue. The proportions of responsive and non-responsive cells in the matrix will ultimately determine the overall responsiveness of the tumour. Even if a tumour initially responds to antioestrogen therapy, the growth of the non-responsive tumour cells will eventually provide enough growth factors to encourage replication of tamoxifen-blocked cells in G1. Measures to discourage this process (strategies to destroy receptor-negative tumour cells or specifically block growth factor action) must be a priority for future research.

Tamoxifen Dependent Growth

The classic study conducted by Dr. Basil Stoll demonstrated that high-dose diethylstilboestrol therapy can initially cause breast tumour regression but then when the tumour starts to grow during therapy, a second response can occur when treatment is withdrawn. Tumour growth appeared to be dependent upon the oestrogen therapy [38].

Tamoxifen does exhibit some oestrogen-like actions in animals and patients and it is possible that tumours can be stimulated to grow with this antioestrogen. Indeed breast cancer cells can be stimulated to grow with low concentrations of antioestrogens in cell culture [39].

There are currently few data in the clinics to support the hypothesis that tamoxifen-dependent growth occurs routinely. This in part may be because tamoxifen has a long biological half-life and requires several months to be cleared from the blood. An early withdrawal response may be difficult to demonstrate. However, there is an anecdotal report of a withdrawal response with tamoxifen [40] and laboratory studies have shown tamoxifen-dependent growth of human tumours in athymic mice. Satyaswaroop [41,42] was the first to demonstrate tamoxifen-stimulated growth of transplanted, oestradiol-dependent, endometrial tumours in athymic mice. The tumour (EnCa101) has oestrogen and progesterone receptors. Athymic mice bitransplanted with breast tumours (MCF-7) and EnCa101 show a target site specificity to tamoxifen therapy. The breast tumour does not grow and tamoxifen inhibits oestradiol-stimulated growth whereas, in the same animal, tamoxifen and oestradiol stimulate endometrial tumour growth [43].

These data suggest that physicians should remain vigilant during long-term adjuvant tamoxifen therapy for the activation of occult uterine carcinoma. It must be stressed though that there have been no reports of increases in endometrial carcinoma as a consequence of the current fashion of adjuvant tamoxifen therapy.

Summary

The development of tamoxifen [44] has provided a valuable non-toxic therapy to control the growth of breast cancer. The successful transfer of the concept that tamoxifen is a tumoristatic therapy from the laboratory to the clinic [5] has provided a useful strategy for the long-term control of disease recurrence in stage I/II breast cancer. Additional treatment strategies must build upon this success to confront the mechanisms of therapeutic failure discussed in this chapter.

In the laboratory the athymic mouse model has proved to be useful to study the hormone-dependent growth of breast and endometrial cancer. Tamoxifen-dependent breast tumour growth has just been reported in this model [14]. Nevertheless, the model is less than perfect and further study of the interaction of endocrine agents with the immune systems of the host may eventually restrict the overall usefulness of this approach. A rigorous validation of this model is long overdue before true tamoxifen-stimulated growth can be studied in detail. A reproducible and clinically relevant model of the failure to tamoxifen therapy has proved to be elusive.

Tamoxifen-stimulated growth may be caused by the weak oestrogen-like properties inherent in the molecule [16]. New non-oestrogenic molecules may be one approach, as a second-generation therapy, to achieve successful long-term disease control [45].

REFERENCES

1   Furr BJA and Jordan VC: The pharmacology and clinical uses of tamoxifen. Pharmac and Therap 1984 (25):127-205

2   Jordan VC (ed) Estrogen/Antiestrogen Action and Breast Cancer Therapy. University of Wisconsin Press, Madison 1986

3   Fisher B, Redmond C, Brown A, Fisher ER, Wolmark N, Bowman D, Plotkin D, Wolter J, Barnstein R, Legault-Poisson S, Soffer EA and other NSABP investigators: Adjuvant chemotherapy with and without tamoxifen in the treatment of primary breast cancer: 5-year results from the National Surgical Adjuvant Breast and Bowel Project Trial. J Clin Oncol 1986 (4):459-471

4   Baum M and other members of the Nolvadex Adjuvant Trial Organisation: Controlled trial of tamoxifen as a single adjuvant agent in management of early breast cancer. Lancet 1985 (i):836-840

5   Jordan VC: Long-term adjuvant tamoxifen therapy for breast cancer: therapies and practice. In: DeVita VT, Hellman S and Rosenburg SA (eds) Important Advances in Oncology. JB Lippincott Company, Philadelphia 1989 (in press)

6   Tormey DC and Jordan VC: Long-term tamoxifen adjuvant therapy in node positive breast cancer: a metabolic and pilot clinical study. Breast Cancer Res Treat 1984 (4):297-302

7   Fisher B, Brown A, Wolmark N, Redmond C, Wickerman DL, Wittliff JL, Dimitrov N, Legault-Poisson S, Schipper H, Prager D and other NSABP investigators: Prolonging tamoxifen therapy for primary breast cancer. Ann Int Med 1987 (106):649-654

8   Breast Cancer Trials Committee, Scottish Cancer Trials Office: Adjuvant tamoxifen in the management of operable breast cancer: the Scottish trial. Lancet 1987 (ii):171-175

9   Jordan VC, Collins MM, Rowsby L and Prestwich G: A monohydroxylated metabolite of tamoxifen with potent antiestrogenic activity. J Endocrinol 1977 (75):305-316

10 Kemp JV, Adam HK, Wakeling AE and Slater R: Identification and biological activity of tamoxifen metabolites in human serum. Biochem Pharm 1983 (32):2045-2052

11 Jordan VC, Bain RR, Brown RR, Gosden B and Santos MA: Determination and pharmacology of a new hydroxylated metabolite of tamoxifen observed in patient sera during therapy for advanced breast cancer. Cancer Res 1983 (43):1446-1450

12 Lyman SD and Jordan VC: Metabolism of tamoxifen and its uterotrophic activity. Biochem Pharm 1985 (34):2787-2794

13 Jordan VC and Robinson SP: Species-specific pharmacology of antiestrogens: role of metabolism. Fed Proc 1987 (46):1870-1874

14 Gottardis MM and Jordan VC: Development of tamoxifen-stimulated growth of MCF-7 tumors in athymic mice after long-term antiestrogen administration. Cancer Res 1988 (48):5183-5187

15 Jordan VC, Fritz NF, Tormey DC: Endocrine effects of adjuvant chemotherapy and long-term tamoxifen administration on node-positive patients with breast cancer. Cancer Res 1987 (47):624-630

16 Jordan VC: Biochemical pharmacology of antiestrogen action. Pharm Rev 1984 (36):245-276

17 Berry J, Green BJ and Matheson DS: Modulation of natural killer cell activity by tamoxifen in stage I postmenopausal breast cancer. Eur J Cancer Clin Oncol 1987 (23):517-520

18 Dickson RB and Lippman ME: Estrogenic regulation of growth and polypeptide growth factor secretion in human breast carcinoma. Endocr Rev 1987 (8):29-43

19 Knabbe C, Lippman ME, Wakefield LM, Flanders KL, Kasid A, Derynck R and Dickson RB: Evidence that transforming growth factor ß is a hormonally regulated negative growth factor in human breast cancer cells. Cell 1987 (48):417-428

20 Sutherland RL, Green MD, Hall RE, Reddel RR, Taylor IW: Tamoxifen induces accumulation of MCF-7 human mammary carcinoma cells in the G0/G1 phase of the cell cycle. Eur J Cancer Clin Oncol 1983 (19):307-318

21 Ingle JN, Krook JE, Green SJ, Kubista TP, Everson LK, Ahman DL, Chang MN, Bisel HF, Windschild HE, Twito DI and Pfeife DM: Randomized trial of bilateral oophorectomy versus tamoxifen in premenopausal women with metastatic breast cancer. J Clin Oncol 1986 (4):178-185

22 Buchanan RB, Blamey RW, Durrant KR, Howell A, Paterson AG, Preece PE, Smith DC, Williams CJ and Wilson RG: A randomized comparison of tamoxifen with surgical oophorectomy in premenopausal patients with advanced breast cancer. J Clin Oncol 1986 (4):1326-1330

23 Sawka CA, Pritchard KI, Paterson DJA, Thompson DB, Skelley WE, Myers RE, Mobbs BG, Malkin A and Meakin JW: Role and mechanisms of action of tamoxifen in premenopausal women with metastatic breast cancer. Cancer Res 1986 (46):3152-3156

24 Ravdin PM, Fritz NF, Tormey DC and Jordan VC: Endocrine status of premenopausal node-positive breast cancer patients following adjuvant chemotherapy and long-term tamoxifen. Cancer Res 1988 (48):1026-1029

25 Hissom JR and Moore MR: Progestin effects on growth in the human breast cancer cell line T47D - possible therapeutic implications. Biochem Biophys Res Commun 1987 (145):706-711

26 Pike MC, Henderson BE, Krailo MD, Duke A and Roy S: Breast cancer in young women and the use of oral contraceptives: possible modifying effects of formulation and age of use. Lancet 1983 (ii):926-930

27 Mouridsen HT, Ellemann K, Mattsson W, Palshoff T, Daehnfeldt JL and Rose C: Therapeutic effect of tamoxifen versus tamoxifen combined with medroxyprogesterone acetate in advanced breast cancer in post-menopausal women. Cancer Treat Rep 1979 (63):171-175

28 Robinson SP and Jordan VC: Reversal of the antitumor effects of tamoxifen by progesterone in the 7,12 dimethylbenzanthracene-induced rat mammary carcinoma model. Cancer Res 1987 (47):5386-5390

29 Biswas R and Vonderhaar BK: Role of serum in the prolactin responsiveness of MCF-7 human breast

cancer cells in long-term tissue culture. Cancer Res 1987 (47):3509-3514

30   Dickson RB, McManaway M and Lippman ME: Estrogen-induced growth factors of breast cancer cells partially replace estrogen to promote tumor growth. Science 1986 (232):1540-1543

31   Dickson RB, Kasid A, Huff KK, Bates SE, Knabbe C, Bronzert D, Gelman EP and Lippman ME: Activation of growth factor secretion in tumorigenic states of breast cancer induced by 17ß estradiol and v-ras^H oncogene. Proc Natl Acad Sci USA 1987 (84):837-841

32   Katzenellenbogen BS, Kendra KL, Norman MJ and Berthois Y: Proliferation, hormonal responsiveness and estrogen receptor content of MCF-7 human breast cancer cells grown in the short-term and long-term absence of estrogens. Cancer Res 1987 (47):4355-4360

33   Welshons WV and Jordan VC: Adaptation of estrogen-dependent MCF-7 cells to low estrogen (Phenol red-free) culture. Eur J Cancer Clin Oncol 1987 (23):1935-1939

34   Jordan VC, Robinson SP and Welshons WV: Resistance to antiestrogen therapy. In: Kessel D (ed) Drug Resistance to Anticancer Agents. CRC Press, Boca Raton 1988 (in press)

35   Cormier EM and Jordan VC: Contrasting ability of antiestrogens to inhibit MCF-7 growth stimulated by estradiol or epidermal growth factor. Eur J Cancer Clin Oncol (in press)

36   Koga M and Sutherland RL: Epidermal growth factor partially reverses the inhibitory effects of antiestrogens on T47D human breast cancer cell growth. Biochem Biophys Res Comm 1987 (147):739-745

37   Robinson SP and Jordan VC: Breast cancer: possible paracrine influences in tamoxifen failure. Proc Am Assoc Cancer Res (New Orleans) 1988 abstract 921

38   Stoll BA: Palliation by castration or by hormone administration. In: Stoll BA (ed) Breast Cancer Management: Early and Late. William Heinemann Medical Books Ltd, London 1977 pp 133-146

39   Darbre PD, Curtis S and King RJB: Effects of estradiol and tamoxifen on human breast cancer cells in serum free culture. Cancer Res 1987 (44):2790-2793

40   Legault-Poisson S, Jolivet J, Poisson R, Perretta-Piccoli M and Band PR: Tamoxifen-induced tumor stimulation and withdrawal response. Cancer Treat Rep 1979 (63):1839-1841

41   Satyaswaroop PG, Zaino RJ and Mortel R: Estrogen-like effects of tamoxifen on human endometrial carcinoma transplanted into nude mice. Cancer Res 1984 (44):4006-4010

42   Clark CL and Satyaswaroop PG: Photoaffinity labeling of the progesterone receptor from human endometrial carcinoma. Cancer Res 1985 (45):5417-5420

43   Gottardis MM, Robinson SP, Satyaswaroop PG and Jordan VC: Contrasting actions of tamoxifen on endometrial and breast tumor growth in the athymic mouse. Cancer Res 1988 (48):812-815

44   Jordan VC: The development of tamoxifen for breast cancer therapy: a tribute to the late Arthur L. Walpole. Breast Cancer Res Treat 1988 (11):197-209

45   Wakeling AE and Bowler J: Steroidal pure antioestrogens. J Endocrinol 1987 (112):R7-R10

New Antioestrogens Without Oestrogenic Activity

A.E. Wakeling

Bioscience Department I, ICI Pharmaceuticals, Alderley Park, Macclesfield, Cheshire, United Kingdom

Introduction

'Nolvadex'[*] (tamoxifen, ICI 46474) - induced regression of breast tumours is conventionally ascribed to the antioestrogenic activity of the molecule. Competition of tamoxifen with endogenous oestrogen for binding to oestrogen receptors in the tumour cells attenuates the proliferative action of oestrogens [1,2]. A large body of evidence derived from studies of breast cancer cells *in vitro*, and of breast tumours in animals supports this simple hypothesis [3]. There remains, however, considerable doubt about whether receptor blockade provides a sufficient or complete explanation for the antitumour effects of 'Nolvadex' [4]. The assumption implicit in the hypothesis is that the tamoxifen-oestrogen receptor complex is essentially inert. That this is not the case is amply demonstrated in pharmacological studies, which reveal that tamoxifen can express a full range of activities from complete antagonism of oestradiol action to full oestrogen agonist effects in both animals and man [1,5]. This complex pharmacology raises a number of issues of importance to the therapeutic use of antioestrogens and, at a more fundamental level, to our understanding of the mode of action of oestrogens.

Because tamoxifen, and all other antioestrogens examined to date, show mixed agonist/antagonist effects, it is impossible to conclude with certainty that any particular action of the compound is due simply to hormone withdrawal. We do not know if the onset,

completeness or duration of tumour remission can be improved by *complete* oestrogen withdrawal. One consequence of the pharmacological actions of tamoxifen and other nonsteroidal antioestrogens in rodents, is that long-term administration produces abnormalities in the development of the reproductive tract [6]. The occurrence of such effects raises concerns about the unrestricted use of 'Nolvadex' for the treatment of oestrogen-responsive non-malignant disorders of the breast and uterus [7] and, in the absence of further long-term safety studies, the potential for preventative therapy in women at high risk of developing breast cancer [8]. Considerations of this kind led us to initiate, at ICI Pharmaceuticals, a search for novel antioestrogens which would satisfy the pharmacological criteria of pure antagonists. The most important criterion was that such compounds should be capable of blocking *completely* the action of oestrogens in all tissues. An important corollary of such activity would be the complete absence in such molecules of *any* trophic activity in immature or ovariectomised animals. In addition it was considered desirable that such compounds should have a high affinity for the oestrogen receptor to maximise the likelihood of specificity and to optimise the potential efficacy.

Strategic Approach

At the initiation of our search for novel antioestrogens the simplest concept was of a molecule which would bind with high avidity to the cytoplasmic oestrogen receptor without

---

[*] 'Nolvadex' is a trademark, the property of Imperial Chemical Industries PLC.

triggering translocation to the cell nucleus. The absence of structural data on the ligand binding site and of a clear definition of the ligand-driven physicochemical changes in the receptor, which are believed to reveal specific sites for DNA binding, precluded any possibility of targeted drug design.

A more empirical approach was therefore necessary to attempt to identify ligands which would "dock" efficiently at the oestradiol binding site but would be derivatised in a manner likely to interfere with secondary structural changes in the receptor molecule associated with activation. It was also apparent that *in vitro* screening, based on ligand receptor binding or ligand receptor-complex association with DNA, would not distinguish between agonists, partial agonists and antagonists [9]. Similar considerations excluded the use of receptor-positive breast cancer cell lines. The system of choice for testing novel compounds was the 3-day uterotrophic/antiuterotrophic assay in immature rats. This assay is highly sensitive and reproducible and had proved capable of distinguishing readily different degrees of agonist activity [10].

A potential starting point for new chemistry was indicated by studies designed to develop oestradiol derivatives suitable for use in affinity-matrix columns for the purification of oestrogen receptors [11]. This work, in turn, originated from earlier studies to prepare antigens coupled to various positions on the oestradiol molecule, suitable for the genera

tion of highly specific antibodies for oestradiol radioimmunoassay [12]. The key observation from this early literature was that oestradiol analogues containing a long, unbranched alkyl chain at the 7-alpha position retained a high affinity for the oestrogen receptor. It should be noted that in this and other laboratories [13] extensive chemical effort to discover pure antagonists amongst nonsteroidal analogues of the triphenylethylene molecule, or of oestradiol substituted at various positions in the steroid nucleus [14], had been uniformly unsuccessful.

Discovery

Chemical synthesis and screening in the rat uterus assay of a series of relatively simply 7-alkyl analogues of oestradiol quickly proved that such molecules possess interesting biological activity. Among early examples (Table 1) a number of compounds with functional groups attached to oestradiol by a decamethylene bridge showed conventional partial agonist activity. However, the n-butyl analogue 5 produced a complete blockade of the uterotrophic effect of oestradiol and, when administered alone, failed to stimulate the uterus. This result was the first indication that certain 7-substituted oestradiol analogues have the primary characteristic of pure antagonists.

Table 1. Activity of C7-substituted oestradiol analogues in the immature rat uterotrophic/antiuterotrophic assay

C7-Substituent $(CH_2)_{10}R$	Dose (mg/kg s.c.)	% Agonism *	% Antagonism **
1 R = COOH	25	23	30
2 R = CH_2OH	25	28	33
3 R = $CH_2N(C_2H_5)_2$	10	34	41
4 R = $CONH(CH_2)_5COOH$	25	19	33
5 R = $CONH(CH_2)_3CH_3$	25	-3	100

*   Percent agonist   = C-A/B-A x 100
**   Percent antagonist   = B-D/B-A x 100
Where A,B,C and D are uterine weights (mg/100 g body weight) for vehicle alone (arachis oil), oestradiol alone, test compound alone or together with oestradiol, respectively

Compound 5 is a mixture of 7-alpha and 7-beta isomers; separation of the isomers showed that activity resides almost exclusively in the 7-alpha-isomer [15]. Further characterisation showed that among 7-alpha-amides, a linking chain length of 4 to 10 methylene units produces pure antagonists provided that an overall length of 16-18 atoms is maintained by varying the size of the amide function [16]. The pharmacology of the most potent compound of this series ICI 164384, the 7-alpha-N-methyl analogue of compound 5, has been described extensively elsewhere (15,17,18). In summary, ICI 164384 is devoid of oestrogenic activity and blocks completely the trophic activity of exogenous or endogenous oestradiol, and of partial agonist antioestrogens like tamoxifen. Biochemical studies of oestrogen receptor binding [17,19] are consistent with the view that ICI 164384 binds with high affinity to the same site as oestradiol in a competitive manner, but fails to activate DNA binding [19]. This profile of activity conforms closely to the criteria outlined at the inception of the search for pure antioestrogens.

Antitumour Potential

A direct comparison of the antitumour activity of ICI 164384 and tamoxifen in rats bearing dimethylbenzanthracene (DMBA) - induced mammary tumours [15] failed to demonstrate a superior effect of ICI 164384. This was disappointing since previous work had shown that ovariectomy is a more effective treatment than tamoxifen in this model system [20] and ICI 164384 produced a castration-like involution of the uterus in intact female rats [15]. In the latter study ICI 164384 did not affect the function of the hypothalamic-pituitary axis and thus appeared to be selective for peripheral oestrogen receptors [15]. Since factors of pituitary origin, particularly prolactin, are known to play an important role in the growth of DMBA-induced tumours [21], the absence of inhibition by ICI 164384 at this level may explain the lack of correspondence between ovariectomy and the effects of this pure antioestrogen. Prolactin secretion is dependent on oestrogen stimulation and decreases pre-

cipitately in ovariectomised animals. Simple comparisons between the efficacy of tamoxifen and pure antioestrogens in the rat DMBA-model may therefore be misleading. The effects of tamoxifen on the hypothalamic-pituitary axis are complex [1], for example prolactin secretion remains unaffected [22] but appetite and weight gain are inhibited [15]. This effect on growth is characteristic of oestrogens [23] and may contribute indirectly to tumour growth inhibition, since dietary restriction alone inhibits the growth of DMBA-induced tumours [24]. Tumour growth inhibition by tamoxifen may be due to multiple mechanisms involving effects on the host as well as direct actions on the tumour. The effects of ICI 164384 appear to be confined to a more specific direct antitumour action. Furthermore, direct comparative studies of antioestrogen effects on the development of the rat mammary gland have shown that tamoxifen promotes full, oestrogen-like ductal development whereas ICI 164384 failed to promote any elongation of the mammary ducts [25].

The relevance of this complex pharmacology to antitumour activity in patients remains uncertain. However, a peripherally selective pure antioestrogen like ICI 164384 may be particularly useful in premenopausal patients since successful blockade of breast and uterine response to oestrogens in both malignant and non-malignant disease may be achieved *without* functional disturbance of the hypothalamic-pituitary-ovarian axis. The fact that ICI 164384, unlike tamoxifen, is devoid of stimulatory effects on mammary epithelium [25], or on uterine development and subsequent fertility of neonatally-treated rats [18], encourages the view that pure antioestrogens have the potential to provide a safe and efficacious means of broadening the range of therapeutic applications of antioestrogens. It seems likely that the efficacy and side-effect profile of tamoxifen and pure antioestrogens will be different.

Finally, it is clear from the foregoing discussion that the efficacy of pure antioestrogens in breast cancer therapy, particularly in comparison with that of 'Nolvadex', is difficult to predict. Some comparative studies of the effects of tamoxifen and ICI 164384 on the growth of MCF-7 human breast cancer cells may be instructive in this respect. Previous work has shown [17,18] that ICI 164384 is not only much more potent, but also more effective than tamoxifen. Both compounds cause blockade of the cell cycle in early G1 phase [26], but ICI 164384 is more effective in reducing the proportion of cells in the total population which continue to synthesise DNA [27]. Extrapolation to the therapeutic setting would predict an improved antitumour activity but definitive proof of this must await clinical trials with a pure antioestrogen.

REFERENCES

1 Furr BJA and Jordan VC: The pharmacology and clinical uses of tamoxifen. Pharmacol Ther 1984 (25):127-205

2 Jordan VC: Biochemical pharmacology of antiestrogen action. Pharmacol Revs 1984 (36):245-276

3 Jordan VC (ed) Estrogen/Antiestrogen Action and Breast Cancer Therapy. University of Wisconsin Press 1986

4 Nicholson RI: Antioestrogens and breast cancer therapy. In: Furr BJA and Wakeling AE (eds) Pharmacology and Clinical Uses of Inhibitors of Hormone Secretion and Action. Bailliere Tindall, Eastbourne 1987 pp 60-86

5 Wakeling AE: Pharmacology of antioestrogens. In: Furr BJA and Wakeling AE (eds) Pharmacology and Clinical Uses of Inhibitors of Hormone Secretion and Action. Bailliere Tindall, Eastbourne 1987 pp 1-19

6 Tucker MJ, Adam HK and Patterson JS: Tamoxifen. In: Laurence DR, McLean AEM and Weatherall M (eds) Safety Testing of New Drugs. Academic Press, London 1984 pp 125-161

7 Jackson IM, Lowery C: Clinical uses of antiestrogens. In: Furr BJA and Wakeling AE (eds) Pharmacology and Clinical Uses of Inhibitors of Hormone Secretion and Action. Bailliere Tindall, Eastbourne 1987 pp 87-105

8 De Waard F, Wang DY: Epidemiology and prevention: workshop report. Eur J Cancer Clin Oncol 1988 (24):45-48

9 Wakeling AE: Anti-hormones and other steroid analogues. In: Green B and Leake RE (eds) Steroid Hormones - A Practical Approach. IRL Press, Oxford 1987 pp 219-236

10 Wakeling AE, Valcaccia B, Newboult E and Green LR: Non-steroidal antioestrogens-receptor binding and biological response in rat uterus, rat mammary carcinoma and human breast cancer cells. J Steroid Biochem 1984 (20):111-120

11 Bucourt R, Vignau M, Torelli V, Richard-Foy H, Geynet C, Secco-Millet C, Redeuilh G and Baulieu EE: New biospecific adsorbents for the purification of estradiol receptor. J Biol Chem 1978 (253):8221-8228

12 Raynaud JP, Azadian-Boulanger G and Bucourt R: Anticorps specifiques de l'estradiol. J Pharmacol (Paris) 1974 (5):27-40

13 Jones CD, Jevnikar MG, Pike AJ, Peters MK, Black CJ, Thompson AR, Falcone JF and Clemens JA: Antioestrogens 2. Structure-activity studies in a series of 3-aroyl-2-arylbenzo [b] thiophene derivatives leading to [6-hydroxy-2-(4-hydroxyphenyl]benzo[b] thien-3-y] [4-[2-(1-piperidinyl)ethoxy]-phenyl]methanone hydrochloride

14 Kelly PA, Asselin J, Caron MG, Raynaud JP and Labrie F: High inhibitory activity of a new antiestrogen, RU 16117 (11alpha-methoxy ethinyl estradiol), on the development of dimethylbenz(a)anthracene-induced mammary tumours. Cancer Res 1977 (37):76-81

15 Wakeling AE, Bowler J: Biology and mode of action of pure antioestrogens. J Steroid Biochem 1988 (30):141-147

16 Bowler J, Lilley TJ, Pittam JD and Wakeling AE: Novel Steroidal pure antioestrogens. Steroids (in press)

17 Wakeling AE and Bowler J: Steroidal pure antioestrogens. J Endocrinol 1987 (12):R7-R10

18 Wakeling AE and Bowler J: Novel antioestrogens without partial agonist activity. J Steroid Biochem 1988 (in press)

19 Weatherhill PJ, Wilson APM, Nicholson RI, Davies P and Wakeling AE: Interaction of the antioestrogen ICI 164,384 with the oestrogen receptor. J Steroid Biochem 1988 (30):263-266

20 Wakeling AE and Valcaccia B: Antioestrogenic and antitumour activities of a series of nonsteroidal antioestrogens. J Endocrinol 1983 (99):454-464

21 Arafah BM, Manni A and Pearson OH: Effect of hypophysectomy and hormone replacement on hormone receptors levels and the growth of 7,12 dimethylbenz(a)anthracene induced mammary tumours in the rat. Endocrinol 1980 (107):1364-1369

22 Jordan VC and Koerner S: Tamoxifen as an antitumour agent: role of oestradiol and prolactin. J Endocrinol 1976 (68):305-311

23 Roy EJ, Maass CA and Wade GN: Central action and a species comparison of the estrogenic effects of an antioestrogen on eating and body weight. Physiol Behav 1977 (18):137-140

24 Schoenarberger H, Kranzfelder G, Hoffmann E, Egginger G, Schmitt H and Taneja AK: Experimentelle chemotherapie des mammakrebses. Pharmazie 1976 (31):590-597

25 Nicholson RI, Gotting KE, Gee J and Walker KJ: Actions of oestrogens and antioestrogens on rat mammary gland development: relevance to breast cancer prevention. J Steroid Biochem 1988 (30):95-103

26 Musgrove EA, Wakeling AE and Sutherland RL: Inhibition of proliferation of MCF-7 human breast cancer cells: similar points of action within the cell cycle of both steroidal and nonsteroidal estrogen antagonists and a calmodulin antagonist. Cancer Res (in press)

27 Wakeling AE, Newboult E and Peters SW: Effects of antioestrogens on the proliferation of MCF-7 human breast cancer cells. J Molec Endocrinol ((in press)

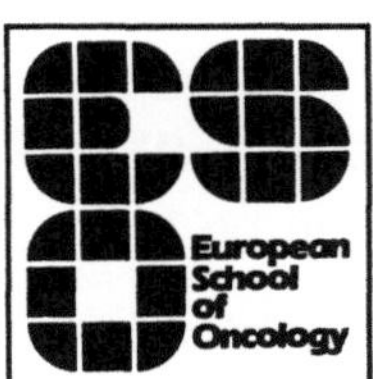

ESO Monographs

Series Editor: U. Veronesi

J.F. Smyth, Edinburgh (Ed.)

Interferons in Oncology

Current Status and Future Directions

1987. VII, 70 pages. Hard cover. ISBN 3-540-18019-2

This monograph summarizes the latest knowledge of the clinical application of interferons in malignant disease with emphasis on hairy cell leukaemia, lymphoma, multiple myeloma, chronic myloid leukaemia, lung cancer, melanoma and renal carcinoma.

L. Domellöf, Örebro (Ed.)

Drug Delivery in Cancer Treatment

1987. VII, 99 pages. Hard cover. ISBN 3-540-18459-7

The authors provide a detailed update of basic and clinical research of drug delivery in cancer treatment, with special reference to pain relief, nutritional support and treatment with anticancer agents. New trends and developments in cancer chemotherapy complete this highly topical monograph.

A.B. Miller, Toronto (Ed.)

Diet and the Aetiology of Cancer

1989. 2 figures. VII, 73 pages. Hard cover. ISBN 3-540-50681-0

L. Domellöf, Örebro (Ed.)

The Role of Drug Delivery in the Supportive Care of Cancer Patients

1989. Hard cover in preparation. ISBN 3-540-51055-9

A. Breit, Munich (Ed.)

Nuclear Magnetic Resonance

1989. Hard cover in preparation. ISBN 3-540-51054-0

Springer-Verlag Berlin
Heidelberg New York London
Paris Tokyo Hong Kong

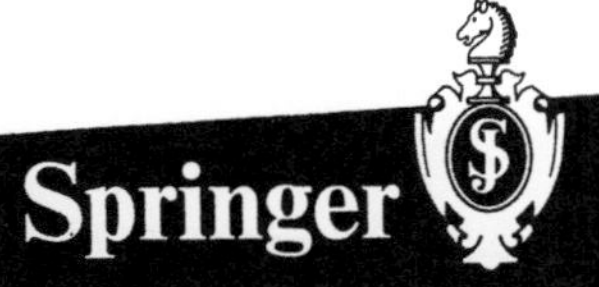

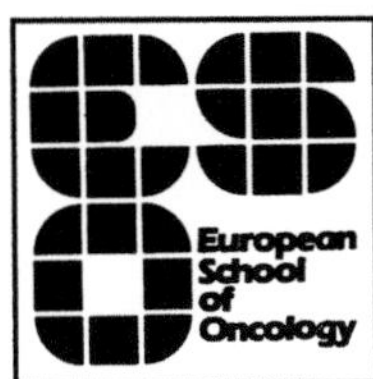

ESO Monographs

Series Editor: U. Veronesi

L. Denis, Antwerp (Ed.)

The Medical Management of Prostate Cancer

1988. 8 figures. IX, 98 pages. Hard cover. ISBN 3-540-18627-1

Contents: Introduction. – Aspects of Epidemiology. Pathogenesis and Natural History of Prostatic Cancer. – Oncogenes, Tumor Markers and Monoclonal Antibodies. – The Endocrinological Basis for Hormonal Therapy. – Estrogens and Estramustine Phosphate. – Antiandrogens. – Luteinizing Hormone Releasing Hormone Agonists. – Chemical Adrenal Blockade Treatment. – Total Androgen Blockade. – Second-Line Endocrine Treatment. – Chemotherapy. – The Clinical and Financial Implications of Immediate or Deferred Treatment in Patients with Advanced Prostatic Cancer. – Treatment Recommendations for Daily Practice.

B. Winograd, Amsterdam; **M. Peckham,** London; **H. M. Pinedo,** Amsterdam (Eds.)

Human Tumour Xenografts in Anticancer Drug Development

1988. 37 figures. XV, 143 pages. Hard cover. ISBN 3-540-18638-7

This monograph covers the latest information on the role of human tumour xenografts in the development of anticancer drugs.
This model has been used in various experimental studies on human tumour morphology, biology, biochemistry and antitumour therapy. Since each individual tumour largely retains its characteristics through serial transplantation in the immune-deficient mouse, this model proves to be particularly valuable in the development of anticancer drugs.

F. Cavalli, Bellinzona (Ed.)

Endocrine Therapy of Breast Cancer

Concepts and Strategies

1986. VII, 120 pages. Hard cover. ISBN 3-540-16959-8

F. Cavalli, Bellinzona (Ed.)

Endocrine Therapy of Breast Cancer III

1989. 26 figures, 7 tables. Approx. 70 pages. Hard cover. ISBN 3-540-50819-8

Springer-Verlag Berlin
Heidelberg New York London
Paris Tokyo Hong Kong

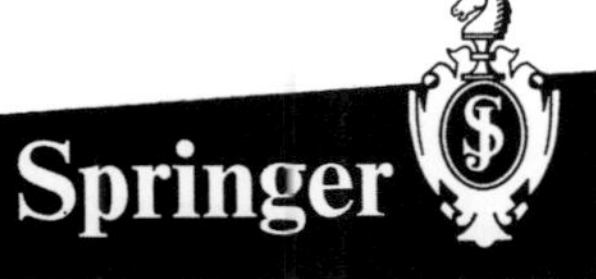